THE EVERYTHING.

Krav Maga for Fitness Book

Dear Reader,

Krav Maga is more than just a system of fighting. While it is one of the hottest forms of fitness currently available, it is more than that as well. Krav Maga is the art of living, offering those who practice it a newfound sense of confidence, the highest level of physical conditioning, and a sense of accomplishment. Krav Maga is a life-altering practice, one that creates athletes and warriors of the highest caliber.

This book provides you with all the tools you need to begin, as well as continue, your journey along the path that is Krav Maga. This book is an all-inclusive training guide that provides more than just basic step-by-step instructions (though these are included) for techniques. Training for fitness requires far more than this. Not just a guide to Krav Maga techniques, this book also offers dietary and nutrition advice, tips for stretching, plus a number of commonly used cross-training practices, such as yoga and kickboxing.

By following this guide, your fitness will improve on a number of levels—cardio, fat burning, energy, and flexibility. The program outlined in this book is not a fad, and it is not a theory. Krav Maga for fitness works…we KNOW it does. And it is our sincere wish that you give it a chance to work for you.

Jeff Levine
Tina Angelotti
Nathan Brown

The EVERYTHING® Series

Editorial

Innovation Director	Paula Munier
Editorial Director	Laura M. Daly
Executive Editor, Series Books	Brielle K. Matson
Associate Copy Chief	Sheila Zwiebel
Acquisitions Editor	Kerry Smith
Development Editor	Brett Palana-Shanahan
Production Editor	Casey Ebert

Production

Director of Manufacturing	Susan Beale
Production Project Manager	Michelle Roy Kelly
Prepress	Erick DaCosta Matt LeBlanc
Interior Layout	Heather Barrett Brewster Brownville Colleen Cunningham Jennifer Oliveira
Cover Design	Erin Alexander Stephanie Chrusz Frank Rivera

THE
EVERYTHING®
KRAV MAGA
FOR
FITNESS
BOOK

Get fit with this high-intensity
martial arts workout!

Jeff Levine and Tina Angelotti with Nathan Robert Brown

Technical Review by Karen West, N.A.S.M., A.C.S.M.

Foreword by Krav Maga Worldwide

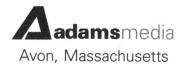

Avon, Massachusetts

An Everything® Series Book.
Everything® and everything.com® are registered trademarks of F+W Publications, Inc.

Published by Adams Media, an F+W Publications Company
57 Littlefield Street, Avon, MA 02322 U.S.A.
www.adamsmedia.com

ISBN 10: 1-59869-424-3
ISBN 13: 978-1-59869-424-6

Printed in the United States of America.

J   I   H   G   F   E   D   C   B   A

Library of Congress Cataloging-in-Publication Data

Levine, Jeff.
The everything krav maga for fitness book / Jeff Levine and Tina Angelotti with Nathan Robert Brown.
p. cm. – (An everything series book)
Includes index.
ISBN-13: 978-1-59869-424-6 (pbk.)
ISBN-10: 1-59869-424-3 (pbk.)
1. Krav maga. 2. Martial arts–Training. I. Brown, Nathan Robert. II.
Levine, Jeff. III. Title. IV. Title: Krav maga for fitness book.
GV1111.A54 2007
796.81–dc22

2007018984

Cover Photographs by Andy Mogg, *www.dancingimages.com*.
Interior photographs by Rodolfo Gonzalez.

This book is available at quantity discounts for bulk purchases.
For information, please call 1-800-289-0963.

CONTENTS

ACKNOWLEDGMENTS

I would like to thank, first and foremost, Tina Angelotti. Without her amazing expertise, this book would not have been possible. I would also like to thank Kerry Smith for all her patience and Jacky Sachs for all of her hard work. Thank you to Adams Media, BookEnds, my family, and to the Graduate staff at Midwestern State University, for putting up with me on those days when I was burned out.

This book is for my mother, Linda Brown. Without her, I never would have made it this far. Also to my daughter, Faith, the greatest teacher I've ever had, and her wonderful mother, Amanda, whom I will always be grateful for.

—Nathan Brown

Top Ten Benefits of
Krav Maga for Fitness

1. You will feel strong and energetic, but you won't look bulky or unnatural.

2. You will create long, lean muscles.

3. You will learn how to burn more calories and fat during your workouts.

4. You will want to move more than you'll want to sit on the couch and watch TV.

5. You will increase your functional strength so everday movements will not lead to injuries.

6. You will form the base for self-defense training.

7. You will learn how to eat for health and fitness.

8. You will learn how to work with your body as it ages, rather than giving in to the erroneous belief that the body has to disintegrate as you get older.

9. You will find balance in your life, and it will include activity and rest, and high-intensity movement and relaxing movement.

10. You will look in the mirror and like what you see.

FOREWORD

Krav Maga is an aggressive, hard-core self-defense system...but fitness has always been a major component of it. One of the first books about Krav Maga, *Fighting Fit* by David Ben-Asher, was focused on the idea of physical fitness. Sheiki Barak, now retired from the Israeli Defense Force, not only has the honor of being the Krav Maga instructor who achieved the highest rank in the Israeli Defense Force (Lieutenant Colonel), he was also in charge of all physical fitness for the IDF. Amir Perets, who is very active with the Krav Maga Worldwide organization in the United States, served as the main instructor in both hand-to-hand combat and conditioning for the IDF's version of the U.S. Navy SEALs.

In the United States, Krav Maga Worldwide (and its godparent, the Krav Maga Association of America) has taken that fitness training to a whole new level. And yet, it's a level easily reached by the average person. This is important because Krav Maga's *raison d'etre* is to be useful to everyone, not just top athletes.

The Krav Maga National Training Center in Los Angeles, California, has 2,000 active members. Most of them come for the self-defense training, but once they join they find one of the most active, vibrant, and satisfying fitness programs available anywhere in the world. This program was initiated by some of Krav Maga's top instructors, including Michael Margolin, a 4th Degree Black Belt in Krav Maga. Over the years, it has been refined and expanded by Tina Angelotti, one of the authors of this book and the person largely responsible for the current success of the Krav Maga fitness program.

The students who take fitness classes at Krav Maga Worldwide's facilities have two things in common. First, they want to become stronger and fitter; and second, they want a workout that is both interesting and practical. Krav Maga's fitness training provides a program that fulfills both those desires. Krav Maga strength is functional strength – using all the right muscle groups to lift, pull, or carry. Krav Maga stamina is functional stamina – your ability to work efficiently over long periods and explosively in short bursts. People who train at Krav Maga Worldwide facilities find themselves looking and (more importantly) feeling leaner, longer, and stronger.

It remains to be said that this is a fitness book, not a self-defense book. It won't teach you to protect yourself against a violent attack. But the exercises in this book *are* designed to complement and reinforce the movements you will learn in a Krav Maga self defense class. So if you bought this book expecting to be a ninja by the last page, stop reading now. But if you started reading because you're looking for practical, functional conditioning that will make you leaner and stronger, and set you up for self defense training, read on: you've come to the right place.

Krav Maga Worldwide

INTRODUCTION

▶ CREATED ON THE VIOLENT STREETS of pre-WWII Europe and developed on the battlefields of the Middle East in an environment where one had little time to devote to combat training, the Krav Maga system was created to bring students to an efficient level of fighting ability in a short period of time. Since its birth, Krav Maga has proven its efficient applicability in the real and violent worlds of war, law enforcement, and civilian "street-wise" self-defense. Changing with the times, Krav Maga has continued to be developed and improved for over a half-century. You will find no specific "forms" (referred to as *kata* in Japanese Martial Arts) in this system, and very few absolute rules (if any). In Krav Maga training, the focus is on **you**. The training in this book is meant to help you develop a high level of physical fitness while teaching you easy-to-learn self-defense techniques that are designed to be effective in reality-based situations of aggression and/or violence.

The path of Krav Maga is far more than just a way of fighting, it is a survival system meant to ensure the practitioner's personal safety. Considered a modern and constantly evolving street fighting system, Krav Maga is effective for use against both armed and unarmed attackers, addressing a variety of potential situations such as defense against punches, kicks, chokes, physical restraints/grabs. What's more, these defenses are learned in such a way that they may be employed against one or multiple attackers, armed with firearms, edged weapons, or blunt objects.

Krav Maga training places emphasis on conditioning oneself to react when caught off-guard. The techniques and training methods will sharpen your ability to defend and counter from a state of non-readiness, teaching you to transition from passive to aggressive modes in the blink of an eye. The training methods will tone your body while teaching you to fight effectively in moments of chaos and stress. The techniques will allow you to learn how to move from a disadvantaged situation to a position of advantage in combative situations.

In addition to self-defense, Krav Maga will harden, strengthen, and lengthen the muscles of your body. You will grow faster, stronger, and more toned with every passing week of training. The training will introduce you to elements that are applicable to the act of fighting—fighting strategies, feints, punching/kicking combinations, blocks, and counterattacks. Psychologically, your confidence and assertiveness will grow as you learn to control fear, to face uncertainty, to remain calm in the midst of chaos, and to use the environment to your advantage.

Krav Maga offers a fitness program that includes specialized training methods that will not only challenge you on a physical level, but will also develop within you a rare mental discipline that will strengthen your spirit and develop your ability to deal with violent encounters under great amounts of mental stress. This is perhaps why so many law enforcement organizations have begun to integrate Krav Maga into their training programs.

Krav Maga is not a combat sport, and you will find no Krav Maga-sanctioned competitions or tournaments. This is not a sport…it is a way to develop the mental acuity and physical strength that will allow you to live and survive in today's harsh world.

The Krav Maga symbol, as seen in the KMAA logo on the cover of this book, consists of a combination of the Hebrew letters K and M surrounded by an open circle. The open circle is symbolic of how the Krav Maga system remains open and constantly evolving, as practitioners are always improving, revising, and adding upon techniques, exercises, and training methods.

1

WHAT IS KRAV MAGA?

The first question most people have when they hear the words *Krav Maga* is, "What's that?" The standard answer is that Krav Maga is the martial art and fighting system of the Israeli Defense Force. However, as you will see, Krav Maga is far more, and its benefits reach far outside the borders of its home of origin in Israel. Krav Maga has extended into the worlds of professional sports, mixed martial arts, and aerobic fitness.

A History of Contact Combat

Krav Maga was originally developed in Israel during the 1940s and 1950s by Imi Lichtenfeld (also known as Imrich Sde-Or) for the Israeli military. Though he was born in Hungary, Lichtenfeld was raised in Bratislava, the largest city and state capital of Slovakia. He excelled in athletics, especially combat sports, earning a number of awards in both wrestling and boxing.

FACT

Imi Lichtenfeld is also known as Imrich Sde-Or (meaning "Light Field," which is a translation of his name into Hebrew) and is the founder of the Krav Maga fighting system. Originally, Lichtenfeld developed Krav Maga as a system of close combat for the Israeli military, or the Israeli Defense Force (IDF).

Imi was the son of a police officer, Samuel Lichtenfeld. Imi's father served for some thirty years as chief inspector and became renowned for his extensive arrest record and for having dealt with a number of dangerous criminals. While on the force, Imi's father owned and operated the Hercules gym in Bratislava where he taught self-defense—constantly focusing his teachings to instruct fellow officers on the importance of moral conduct with the public and the proper treatment of suspects during detainment.

On the Streets of Bratislava

It was on the streets of Bratislava that Imi Lichtenfeld developed and sharpened his fighting ability, birthing what would later come to be known as Krav Maga. Originally, Imi's motivations were to protect himself and his Jewish neighbors from the anti-Semitic violence of local fascist gangs. In order to protect his community, Imi would often have to fight these men (some of whom were armed) with only his hands.

During this time Imi began to reflect on the combat sports of his past. From these experiences, he became aware of the basic differences between combat sports and fighting on the mean streets of reality. This principle would later become the foundation of Krav Maga.

Imi's home was turned into a battlefield during the late 1930s as Hitler's Nazi Germany turned Europe into a hunting ground for Jews. Imi's strength and his efforts to protect his community made him a target of the Nazi Party. By 1940, Imi had no choice but to flee his home. Following years of travel, he settled in what was then Palestine and is now modern-day Israel.

Shortly after settling in Israel, Imi joined a paramilitary Jewish organization known as the Haganah and joined the fight for an independent state of Israel. It was during this time that he began teaching the basics of hand-to-hand and close combat to his fellow soldiers.

Krav Maga's Development in Israel

When the sovereign state of Israel was officially formed in 1948, the government contracted Imi to develop a system of hand-to-hand combat for soldiers, which would come to be called Krav Maga.

When the Haganah was merged into the Israeli Defense Force (IDF), Imi was appointed Chief Instructor of Physical Training and Krav Maga at the Israeli military's training facility.

QUESTION

What does Krav Maga mean?
Krav Maga is Hebrew for "contact combat." Today, soldiers and law enforcement officials all over the world study Krav Maga as a form of close combat and nonlethal suspect management. It is also growing in popularity as a form of physical fitness.

For twenty years, Imi continued to serve in the Israeli Defense Force, further developing his Krav Maga system as he trained both soldiers and instructors for the most elite military units in the country. The object of such a fighting system was, in fact, to remove the system by sacrificing ideas such as fixed positions and right and wrong mentalities for natural and efficient reactions that worked. The main idea was to create a fighting system that could be quickly learned, practiced, and effectively put into use by men and women who had little or no previous fighting experience, regardless of their size or strength. It needed to be quickly learned and easily retained with minimum practice.

In order for this to be achieved, Krav Maga focuses on what has proven to be effective in combat. Krav Maga is not a martial art of theory but one of practice.

Israel was in a constant state of war with its neighboring countries throughout the 1950s and 1960s, and continues to have conflicts with its neighbors even today. Due to this, the techniques of Krav Maga have been tirelessly tested for decades. Each technique was proven either effective or useless in the real-world combat on the battlegrounds of the Middle East.

Imi's Idea of Retirement

By 1964 Imi Lichtenfeld had retired from active duty. Never one to become complacent, he began to redefine a new focus for Krav Maga. This time the battlefields would not be that of soldiers but the violent, unexpected situations that confronted ordinary citizens in everyday life. Imi now decided to teach his system to civilians in Israel. He modified the system of Krav Maga so that ordinary people who lead ordinary lives could employ it.

Krav Maga became popular among Israeli civilians very quickly as teams of instructors, intensively trained by Imi himself, spread it all over the country. Imi himself handpicked each of these instructors, and Imi, as well as the Israeli Ministry of Education, accredited all of them as teachers of Krav Maga.

3

The Rise of Krav Maga

As a military fighting system, Krav Maga is tested every day both in Israel and in the United States. Krav Maga was introduced to the United States over twenty years ago by Darren Levine, chief Krav Maga instructor in the United States, and it has only continued to gain in popularity. Levine holds one of only two Krav Maga Founder's Certificates and is one of only two sixth-degree Krav Maga black belts in the world.

FACT

In 1984 Darren Levine became the first American to receive a Full Instructor Certification in Krav Maga. After attending the First International Instructor's Course in Krav Maga, he became a friend and student of Imi Lichtenfeld. He is also responsible for bringing Krav Maga to the United States from Israel.

In 1981, Levine attended the First International Instructor's Course held at the Wingate Institute in Israel by the Krav Maga Association of Israel. Levine was one of only twenty-three members from the United States who were sponsored (by philanthropist S. D. Abraham) to attend the event. At seventy-one years of age, Imi Lichtenfeld was still able to effectively supervise the six-week course himself.

Enter Darren Levine

As a result of his martial arts and boxing experience (along with his role in the physical education program of the Heschel Day School near Los Angeles, California), Levine was among the few selected to attend. During the exhausting eight-hour-a-day, six-week-long training program, Imi and Levine developed a friendship. Before Levine left Israel, Imi told him that he would come to the United States the next summer to train him personally.

In the summer of 1982, Imi made good on his promise. He came to Los Angeles for several weeks, spending time with Levine and his family while instructing him further in Krav Maga. This training would become a yearly tradition. Every summer after that, either Levine would go to Israel or Imi (or one of his top instructors) would come to the United States for training.

Levine Brings Krav Maga to School

After his 1981 trip, Levine began teaching Krav Maga as an elective at the Los Angeles school where he ran the physical education program. Krav Maga soon became so popular that it was permanently incorporated as a part of the physical education program.

In addition to being a Kravist and a teacher, Levine played another important role—that of Deputy District Attorney in L.A. County. As a result, Levine regularly prosecuted offenders for violent crimes made against police officers. This unique position allowed Levine the opportunity to evaluate and analyze situations in his prosecution arguments, as well as recreate violent encounters for juries in the courtroom. This position also gave him the unique opportunity to constantly review and test the effectiveness of certain Krav Maga (and other) fighting techniques in close combat on the street and to make changes based on what he had learned.

ESSENTIAL

A Kravist is a practitioner of Krav Maga. No one is certain when or where this term came into use, and some schools of Krav Maga do not use it at all. Some speculate that this term started being used by westerners who had previous traditional martial arts backgrounds.

In 1984, at the ceremony for Levine's first-degree black belt in Krav Maga, Imi Lichtenfeld passed on his own black belt to his close friend and student. At this ceremony, Levine became the first American to receive a Full Instructor Certification in Krav Maga from the Wingate Institute for Physical Education and Sports as well as the Krav Maga Association of Israel.

Krav Maga Comes to the United States

In 1987, Krav Maga was introduced to the United States law enforcement community. Under the supervision of Imi, Levine and his students began adapting Krav Maga in ways that would suit the special needs of U.S. law enforcement personnel as well as members of the military. The Illinois State Police would be the first law enforcement agency to officially adopt Krav Maga as part of its curriculum. Imi, now seventy-seven years old, flew to the United States to observe the course. This was only the beginning for Krav Maga in the United States.

Over the last twenty years, Krav Maga has grown to become one of the most highly regarded self-defense and reality-based fighting systems in the world. Today Krav Maga is taught to over 350 U.S. law enforcement organizations, including the FBI, CIA, Federal Air Marshals Service, Los Angeles County Sheriff's Department, U.S. Immigrations and Customs Enforcement (ICE), U.S. Secret Service, the United States Army, the United States Air Force, the United States Marine Corps, and the United States Navy.

Krav Maga's Place in the Martial Arts World

One way in which Krav Maga differs from some of the more traditional martial arts is that Krav Maga focuses on the "martial" part, and changes are made to the system whenever it makes sense to do so.

There is an ongoing debate among Kravists about the best techniques. With little emphasis on having a fixed "art," so-to-speak, Kravists have little difficulty discarding any technique as long as there is something that better serves the practitioner's specific needs, purposes, and/or principles. They therefore acknowledge that combative situations, like life, are never exactly the same.

The perfect fighting system would be one that has only one very simple but effective technique that works against every single attacker, every single time. The problem is that every attacker, environment, situation, and the standard of what is considered an appropriate use of force will not always be the same. As a result, no single technique will work every time for every attacker in every situation.

The Mindset of Krav Maga

Krav Maga, as a system, encompasses self-defense as well as offensive hand-to-hand combat techniques against both armed and unarmed attackers. The training is designed to offer simulated situations that are as close to the real thing as can be safely practiced.

Along with the physical skills, Krav Maga training develops your ability to control your aggression on an emotional level, meaning that it will train you to release your aggression in controlled bursts when and if needed.

Since the majority of people are not familiar with Krav Maga, the easiest way to explain it is to compare it with other more commonly known martial arts. Most martial arts come from the countries of the Far East and are the result of thousands of years of spiritual and historical tradition. However, they all stem from a common thread—the need to defend oneself, one's country, or one's family from a perceived threat.

Not Your Grandfather's Karate!

The people of Okinawa, a small island off the coast of Japan, first developed what is now known as karate in response to being forbidden to carry weapons by the ruling samurai class. However, it was a violent world, and the Shuri-te bodyguards of Okinawa's royal family had to face that world unarmed.

ESSENTIAL

While Krav Maga emphasizes aggressive responses to violent situations, this should not be mistaken for blind rage. The strikes and counters of the system, while aggressive and rapid, are not just blind flurries thrown with anger. Control is a primary principle of Krav Maga training.

To make matters worse, the Okinawan people were charged with the responsibility of keeping any and all foreign naval vessels off of their island, an unbending law that was set upon them by a military dictatorship. They were ordered to turn back all foreign sailors at the shore and they had to do so without the benefit of weaponry.

If It Works, Use it!

Similar to the situation surrounding the founding of karate, Krav Maga was created from a survivalist situation in which it needed to work. While some of the older, more traditional martial arts, such as karate, are now studied as a way of preserving certain martial traditions of the past, Krav Maga is less of a tradition and far more a constantly evolving system meant for use in combat.

The Krav Maga system is not set in stone because all things change. Nothing ever stays the same forever. Krav Maga is designed to be effective in an ever-changing and sometimes violent world.

The Rise of MMA and NHB in America

Most recently, the emerging popularity of no-holds-barred (NHB) and mixed martial arts (MMA) gyms, reality shows, and competitions—such as the Lion's Den Gym, the reality show *The Ultimate Fighter*, and the popular Ultimate Fighting Championship (UFC)—have done a lot to increase interest and awareness among the general public.

In contrast to what is often portrayed in today's action and martial arts films, few one-on-one fights last more than thirty seconds. The reason for this is simple—both people may attack, but usually it only takes one person connecting one blow to one target in order to end a fight.

In professional fights, the length of the encounter depends upon the fighting styles, physical fitness, amount of training, past experiences, and skill levels of one or both fighters. These fights tend to have a wide range of possible time durations, lasting anywhere from just a few seconds to as long as an hour or more.

In the MMA/NHB ring there are often rules in place to reduce the risk of fighters suffering permanent damage such as blindness, infections, or even paralysis.

There are few rules in MMA/NHB, and the most common are no biting, no hair pulling, no attacks to the neck/throat, kneecaps, or groin, and no eye gouging. Aside from these targets, next to nothing is taboo, leaving fighters with a broad range of combative and strategic possibilities.

In a real-world situation, one attacker can become two or more very quickly, and they rarely have any qualms about attacking the vital areas of your body that could permanently damage, paralyze, or even kill you. While Krav Maga training will definitely increase your odds of being able to win (or at the very least survive) a one-on-one confrontation, such training will also teach you the tools and endurance needed to defend against multiple attackers.

Krav Maga's Emphasis on Conditioning

Anyone who has ever fought, competitively or on the streets, will tell you that when you're fighting an opponent, even thirty seconds can seem like a *very* long time. Why? The answer is simple: In a fight you have to put everything you have physically against everything your opponent has. The fighter who has more to give (both in mind and body) has the advantage. The first fighter to run out of steam or lose confidence is likely the first one to be knocked out.

Hard Realities

There is a hard reality of fighting—your fitness level has a lot to do with your chances of winning a fight or simply surviving an attack. If Krav Maga is to deliver on its promise to practitioners that they will be able to defend themselves, then it must do what it can, on an individual case-by-case basis, to address every Kravist's physical fitness level.

> **FACT**
>
> There are currently about 220 Krav Maga gym locations worldwide: 210 in the United States, 7 in Europe (soon to be 9), 2 in Israel, and 1 in Japan. To find specific locations for a Krav Maga center near you, go to *www .kravmaga.com/locations.asp.*

Krav Maga is a training program for adults, meaning that most practitioners have families, jobs, and other responsibilities. This means that Krav Maga must be able to work for people who have a limited amount of time to devote to training, and there has been more of an interest in the fitness aspects of Krav Maga than on the self-defense benefits.

Harder Than Reality

Krav Maga delivers on its promises as both an excellent physical fitness program as well as a method of self-defense, not to mention that it does so quickly, effectively, and in a fun, empowering, and energizing way. The cardiovascular conditioning gained from Krav Maga training is often far more intense than can be found in many other martial arts program.

Applications to Other Sports

All athletic activities, in one form or another, rely on balance, speed, agility, coordination, power, and reaction. With Krav Maga training, all of these components are implemented into the training sessions. Short bursts of power, quickly changing directions, acceleration, and slowing down: all of these skills will be practiced, some in the form of drills and others directly applied to techniques.

This type of training will enhance the performance of any athlete in any sport or activity. It doesn't matter whether you are looking to improve on a basketball player's jump shot, a baseball player's swing of the bat, a golfer's swing, preparing for a triathlon, or looking to build up your legs for outdoor cycling. Krav Maga can help you to improve both mentally and physically.

The Competitive Edge

No matter the sport, Krav Maga training can give any athlete the competitive edge, on both the physical and mental levels, that is needed in order to win. After a few months of training, you will be able to see and feel the physical improvements that Krav Maga provides. You will then be able to modify your workout to your own individual performance level in a way that applies most directly to your particular training needs in any other sport.

The Mental Edge

Right from the beginning you will begin to develop mental skills that will help you compete in the real world. These skills include a can-do lifestyle and a never-quit attitude. You will develop mastery over your will as well as gain a sharper focus that will allow you to calmly and effectively deal with all kinds of challenges that come your way, not just physical confrontations.

You may also find that you cease to be as easily intimidated. Such a mental attitude embodies the very spirit of Krav Maga and carries as much importance as the physical skills do. At first you might be limited in how far you can develop simply because you cannot see beyond what you believe you are capable. But once you start breaking down these self-imposed mental barriers, you will find you are capable of things that you never dreamed possible.

Krav Maga training techniques and drills are designed in a progressive way that enables you, the student, to recognize where your edge is, what your biggest challenges are, and how to push yourself to the next level in a safe and intelligent manner. And you will find yourself doing so without wasting so much as a moment's thought about being defeated. You will build on your courage, confidence, and perseverance through this training program, and it will begin to translate into every component of your everyday life.

The Ultimate Workout

Every possible component of mind and body fitness is incorporated into a Krav Maga fitness program. The program starts by building a stable foundation within your body for you to work with. The next focus is to build upon your functional strength and to begin to apply that strength to the Krav Maga system or any other sport.

9

Lastly, your training will focus on learning how to develop your power and explosiveness, whether through a vertical jump or a left hook punch. For more specific information on techniques, drills, exercises, and workout routines, please refer to Chapters 13, 14, and 18.

ALERT

Measuring body weight alone is a very limiting way of rating fitness. Muscle weighs more than fat. Just because your weight scale says you weigh the same, it does not mean you are not losing fat. Also, being rail thin does not mean you are healthy or fit. You should focus on your own overall fitness level, not the numbers on a scale.

The Krav Maga fitness program will teach your body how to move through the world with physical grace and a state of mental and emotional ease and awareness. The cardiorespiratory training that is included within the system will increase your body's metabolic rate (see Chapter 4), which will help to decrease your body fat percentage.

The flexibility training aspect will lead to lengthened and more efficient joints and muscles, keeping the body mobile as you age. The strength training component will increase lean body mass as well as promote overall joint and skeletal health. In the long run, any exercise program helps to fight the ailments of aging, but Krav Maga is the only system that can get you into outstanding shape as well as teach you to be safe at the same time.

Getting Results

Krav Maga training simultaneously builds muscular, mental, cardiovascular, and core strength, and it improves flexibility, vision, reaction time, endurance, self-control, speed, and the body's resting metabolic rate while it reduces stress. Krav Maga training is a balanced approach to becoming truly fit and will take you as far as you are willing to go! Dramatic results should be apparent in thirty days, and a drastic change in your physical appearance can be seen in ninety days.

Krav Maga for Everyone

Perhaps the best evidence of the benefits of Krav Maga training can be seen on television and the big screen. And Krav Maga is not a practice that is restricted only to males. Many women enjoy Krav Maga fitness training, and they reap the same benefits as men. Many celebrities have begun Krav Maga training—Jennifer Garner (from TV's *Alias*), Christian Bale (*Batman Begins*), James Gandolfini (from HBO's *The Sopranos*), Jennifer Lopez (*Enough*), and Shannon Elizabeth (*American Pie*)—to name just a handful. In fact, Jennifer Lopez received intensive Krav Maga training to prepare for her role in the movie *Enough*. In the film, Lopez plays a battered wife who chooses not to be a victim and decides that she's not going to be battered anymore. She trains for months and confronts her abusive husband one-on-one using Krav Maga!

In reality, women often thrive under Krav Maga training. So forget all that "it's not ladylike to fight" business! If that were true, then why were you given the ability?

2 GETTING MOTIVATED

One of the hardest obstacles for you to overcome when you start your training will be to stay motivated. This means being motivated not only in the first few weeks but also throughout your Krav Maga training program. Learning about the process of motivation will help get you on the right track. It always helps to find something that you enjoy doing and that you have a keen interest in learning. Krav Maga is always evolving and growing, and for that reason alone it excels at keeping your interest. There is always something more for you to learn, practice, or improve upon.

Training with a Purpose

Krav Maga is considered training with a purpose. You will not see a teacher of Krav Maga asking a student to perform an exercise simply because that teacher said so. Krav Maga is not your old-school karate dojo where questions were often discouraged and could even be considered disrespectful at times. In Krav Maga, you, the student, are welcomed and encouraged to ask questions of instructors and trainers. This way, you will be more capable of fully understanding the concepts and principles that are being introduced during your training.

ESSENTIAL

Motivation is often easy to come by during the first few weeks of your training. However, oftentimes it is tempting to skip a day for the usual reasons. Resist that temptation; you will regret skipping a day! While you may have to force yourself to train every now and then, you will never regret having done so.

Every movement, every drill, and every sequence has a reason and a purpose for why it is being performed. Most of these exercises have more than one purpose. When you can begin to pick out what the specific goal is for performing a certain drill or exercise, it will seem as if the exercise suddenly has depth and substance that you did not see before. The activity then becomes much more engaging to you, and will keep you motivated to continue with your program.

A Reason for Training

The most popular and obvious reason to maintain your training program is to stay in control of your body weight. According to the National Institute of Health (NIH), nearly one-third of all American adults are overweight, many to the point of obesity. Sadly, NIH research also indicates that less than half of the adults in this country are at what is considered a healthy weight. Those who are overweight will often think that all they need to do is diet in order to lose weight. And while dieting does cut down calories and will help shed pounds, exercise is sometimes overlooked. This is why so many dieters find themselves back at square one, gaining back all the weight they lost during a period of dieting. Permanent lifestyle changes, namely diet and fitness, must be implemented in order to maintain a healthy weight.

ALERT

Diets are temporary. Lifestyle changes are more permanent. A diet will, at some point, start to get a little old. Eventually you will get tired of counting calories and carbs. Adopting a lifestyle of a balanced diet and regular exercise is the real key to losing weight and keeping it off. There is no magic diet that works indefinitely and for everyone.

Many people think that exercising will only increase their appetite. This just simply is not true if you are exercising with moderate intensity.

It has been shown that if you perform thirty minutes of cardiorespiratory exercise at least five times a week, you can and often will experience a weight loss of twenty to twenty-five pounds in the first year...but only if your caloric intake remains the same.

QUESTION

What is the secret to losing weight?
There are two ancient secrets to losing weight and looking great—proper diet and regular exercise. Read the fine print on any and all products that make weight-loss claims and you will find that nearly all of them include the words "with regular diet and exercise." Guess what? Just about anything taken or done during a period of diet and exercise could make the same claim.

Another health factor that exercise can have a positive effect on is hypertension, which is high blood pressure. Regular cardiorespiratory exercise has been shown to decrease blood pressure. High blood pressure is a prime risk factor in coronary heart disease. An increase in your systolic blood pressure, up to 150 mmHg, can double your chance of developing heart disease, which is the number one killer in the United States today. Knowing that a small amount of activity can have such a large impact on the insides of your body can help motivate you to keep moving.

At War with Your Emotions

Exercise is also a great way to more effectively deal with the anxiety and stress of our everyday lives. It has been shown that people who are on a regular exercise program have much lower levels of stress and anxiety. Exercise can also increase your self-esteem. The satisfaction and accomplishment of being able to do something you were not able to do before provides a good boost in self-esteem. Lastly, people who exercise feel more confident about the way they look. They usually carry themselves well, have better posture, and walk or move as if they have more energy (primarily because they do).

Many of the exercises that are done in Krav Maga involve a partner. When you have a friend with you, your training session becomes more fun. It gives you a chance to spend time together and socialize. Training with a partner or friend also helps keep both of you on track because you can help each other stay motivated and not fall prey to putting your workout off because you are too tired or busy. Find a friend to train with and work hard to keep one another in check.

The Same Old Excuses

Many people use the excuse that they do not have enough time to exercise. If you take a look at your schedule, this is usually perception rather than reality. Lack of time is not the problem. The problem is making exercise a priority and sticking with it.

13

Personal trainers, coaches, and exercise leaders will usually reinforce the benefits of exercise to keep their clients and athletes motivated to stay on their training program.

When exercise is enjoyable, satisfying, meaningful, and convenient it is likely that it will get done. The Krav Maga training program is convenient due to the fact you can do it in your home, backyard, or gym. It is meaningful in that you are learning something that you may need to use to save your life, and it's a great workout so you will feel satisfied with the time and work you put into your workout session. Lastly, it's an enjoyable and fun workout.

More Excuses!

The second most popular excuse is lack of energy. Busy schedules, and the fatigue that goes with it, are the norm these days. If you pay attention to the fatigue you experience in the middle of the day, you may notice that it's usually mental fatigue rather than physical fatigue, which means it is triggered by stress. Remember that exercise can help alleviate stress. If you take time out of your day to do a thirty- to forty-five-minute workout routine, you may find that the mental fatigue has dissipated and you feel refreshed and energized for the rest of your day.

If you are feeling fatigued, take a few slow, deep breaths in and out. Sit or stand up tall, and as you inhale reach your arms up over your head. As you exhale let your arms come back down by your sides.

Breathing can be very energizing whether you are preparing to workout or sitting at your computer. Abdominal exercises are very energizing as well. If you begin your workout and are feeling sluggish, choose a warm-up that incorporates an abdominal sequence. You will find that you are more energized upon completion.

The last excuse is lack of motivation. It takes commitment and dedication to maintain your training regime. It becomes very easy to put off your workout until tomorrow to meet friends for dinner tonight. Keep in mind the positive benefits of being physically active. Just getting in there and doing it, even when you feel like you don't want to, will remind you of how great you feel when you exercise. When you're feeling undermotivated, commit to just ten or twenty minutes of exercise, then see where that takes you. No matter how long you train, it all starts with just one training session.

ALERT

Leave the stressors of your world outside when you come to train! All the things that stress you out or cause you anxiety will still be there when you are done with your training session, but they probably won't seem as stressful after your workout. Just let yourself be! It is counterproductive for you to worry about calling the plumber to fix a leaky faucet while you are working out. Leave such thoughts at home when you come to train.

There are a few ways to keep yourself motivated to get to your training session. First, it may help to train with a friend. You are not likely cancel if someone else is depending on you, and you are able to hang out with your friend at the same time. Also, staying committed to your workout routine might be a nice opportunity for you to set a good example for a friend or spouse. Try going to a Krav Maga class at your local Krav Maga facility. Training in a room full of other people learning the same thing can be motivating and fun. If that is not possible you may consider working with a personal trainer. That way you have an appointment and you don't have to think as much about what you are going to do. You just show up and they help motivate you through the entire workout. Most Krav Maga training centers offer some kind of personal training or private lessons.

Psychological Health and Well-Being

It is very common these days for doctors to prescribe drugs for anxiety or depression or to suggest treament with psychotherapy. These methods are effective, but exercise can be just as beneficial.

All types of exercise are effective, but it has been shown that the longer the duration of the training bout, the greater the antidepressant effect. Although exercise alone can help, it may be best to combine exercise and psychotherapy to obtain the greatest results.

The Elation of Exercise

Have you ever noticed when you finish an exercise session that you have feelings of satisfaction, happiness, or elation? These feelings or moods can last for hours, sometimes even days. Psychotherapists will say that exercise is an effective technique for changing a bad mood. People who exercise frequently know this well and use this technique to work through their anger, anxiety, or any other emotional state they may be feeling.

As mentioned earlier, regular exercise enhances one's body image, thus enhancing self-esteem. It has been found that individuals with low self-esteem, and even individuals who have no problems with low self-esteem, are affected by this phenomenon. When it comes to children, positive changes in self-esteem have been associated with the involvement of physical education classes and after-school programs where sports and physical activity are emphasized. If it's possible to begin this behavior in children, it is likely they will continue with this throughout their lifespan.

How and Why Does This Phenomenon Occur?

There are several ideas or theories to explain why exercise enhances psychological well-being. Unfortunately, there is not one theory that has enough support as the primary mechanism for causing these changes. On a physiological level, there is an increase of blood flow to the tissues of the brain.

15

This increase in blood flow also results in an increase in oxygen consumption to these tissues, which may create a sense of euphoria. Another explanation is that there are changes in the brain's neurotransmitters so hormones such as epinephrine, norepinephrine, and serotonin (feel-good hormones) have a more powerful effect on the brain and human emotions.

Other Psychological Changes

Individuals who are on a consistent training program report feeling an improvement in imagination, greater feeling of control, and greater feelings of self-sufficiency. In some cases it was found that positive changes in personality adjustments occurred. For example, you may become less irritable.

When the kids are pulling at your shirt or your significant other is doing something her way instead of your way, these are little triggers that affect your state of mind and well-being. You are more likely to brush it off and be a more enjoyable person to be around when you follow a consistent training program.

Know Yourself

Other personality traits that may be enhanced are things such as having a sense of involvement, commitment, and purpose in you daily life. People who feel like they have a purpose, are involved in social clubs and events, or follow through with their commitments to other people usually have a well-developed sense of their self.

The ability to see unexpected changes and challenges that may arise in everyday life as an opportunity rather than another problem can also increase the sense of self.

Exercise is a great way to increase this self-development as well. Exercise keeps energy levels consistent so you have enough endurance to enjoy activities and events. In return, you experience a sense of purpose and involvement, and so on. It becomes a cyclical effect.

ESSENTIAL

Not getting enough sleep is detrimental to training as well as to a healthy lifestyle. The effects of sleep deprivation on your mind and body can include negative symptoms such as increased appetite, weakened immune system, pain sensitivity, headaches, irritability, paranoia, compromised visual acuity, drop in physical endurance, and (of course) fatigue and sleepiness.

Old Notions

For many years teachers and pediatricians assumed that the correct development of movement was important to the development of intelligence in children. Although the research is still inconclusive, the type of training within the Krav Maga system is created to challenge students mentally as well as physically.

The motor skills involved in sending different left and right combinations with your hands or legs requires the nervous system to recall or remember how to do these complex movements in the correct order. Many Krav Maga students have reported an increase in memory after a period of consistent Krav Maga fitness training. Other people have reported being able to think faster on their feet. These are cognitive benefits to exercise.

Movements or exercises that challenge any skill-related components of fitness—such as balance, agility, coordination, speed, power, or reaction time—enhance one's cognitive functioning. For example, hand-eye coordination exercises, such as tossing a medicine ball back and forth, may seem simple.

Try tossing the ball while balancing on one foot. If that still feels simple, have your partner toss the ball at different angles. By incrementally changing a simple exercise, you challenge the nervous system and keep individuals concentrating and focused on their performance. Every time you challenge the nervous system, you are training the brain to think more efficiently.

A Better Lifestyle Means a Better Life

How about lifestyle? When you make training a part of your life, you will start to notice that the quality of your life begins to improve. You will begin to have better sleeping habits. You will find that you are falling asleep faster and that you have an easier time staying asleep throughout the night.

You will start to make better food choices without having to think about or struggle over them. You will begin to exhibit a more positive attitude toward every facet of your life, such as issues at work, and this will allow you to be able to better cope with stress, anxiety, and physical tension. All of these things make for a better quality lifestyle.

The Training High (Runner's High)

There is a phenomenon that can be very addictive among endurance athletes. It is described as a feeling of liberation, perfect rhythm and exhilaration, mental alertness and awareness, and effortless movement. This is commonly known as runner's high. In order to reach this sensation it usually requires rhythmic, long-lasting, and uninterrupted activity.

QUESTION

How do you know if you're experiencing a runner's high?
While many runners have reported experiencing a state of euphoria while running, the actual state they describe varies from one person to the next. When asked to describe this high, athletes commonly call it a state of pleasure experienced after going a certain distance. However, this high isn't solely experienced by runners. Boxers, football players, wrestlers, and even Olympic gymnasts have all reported experiences of euphoria while performing at levels of maximum physical potential.

Although Krav Maga workouts are usually interrupted by changes, a state of euphoria has been experienced by some when music, punching, and kicking are all combined in a rhythmic format. This format is then continued in moderate intensities for long durations. This is similar to a cardio-kickboxing type of class.

Exercise Addicts?

This experience of euphoria and heightened sense of well-being can be addictive. As crazy as it may sound, exercise addiction is a real possibility. While this is probably the least harmful addiction you could ever hope to have, it is often characterized by an experience of withdrawal symptoms within a twenty-three to thirty-six hour period of no physical exercise.

These withdrawal symptoms are usually mild and include irritability, feelings of guilt, twitching of the muscles, feeling bloated, anxiety, and onsets of nervous behaviors (such as compulsive nail-biting and ticking). These behaviors normally only occur if an "addict" is prevented from exercising for any reason for more than a day.

Psychological Effects of an Injury

Unfortunately, injuries happen to even the best athletes. Whether you strain your shoulder while throwing a ball around with the kid next door or turn your ankle while stepping off of a street curb.

It's a hard fact—injuries do occur. When they do, they will limit your exercise routine significantly depending on the extent of your injury.

Though you may not necessarily be addicted to exercise, you may experience some of the same responses as an exercise addict. This is just your body's way of telling you that it has become accustomed to regular exercise. The frustration you may feel often comes from not having a choice in whether you perform physical activity. Irritability, anxiety, low self-esteem, and guilt are just some of the emotions that an injured individual who leads an active lifestyle may feel when forced to curtail physical activity.

Don't Let an Injury Get You Down

No one expects you to walk around saying, "I am so happy that I dislocated my shoulder! How cool is that?" However, it's important to maintain a positive attitude about your injury. It has been discovered by athletic trainers that injuries can heal faster by using combinations of a social support structure, healing imagery exercises, goal setting, and positive self-talk. Athletes should maintain positive behaviors when injured, which will better equip them to handle injuries.

Athletes are more likely to comply with their rehabilitation and treatment processes by staying motivated, dedicated, and determined to heal and get better. Athletes are more likely to ask questions and are therefore often more knowledgeable about their injuries. An injury should be seen as a learning process. If you pay close attention to the effects of the injury, you can learn a lot about yourself and your behaviors.

ALERT

Training through an injury does not make you tough. If anything, it just causes your injury to get even worse and could even lead to permanent damage! Listen to your body and your physician. It's always best to ask your doctor about specific types of exercises you can perform while healing, thus allowing you to stay in shape without upsetting your injury.

Tips for Continuing Your Training Program

Many people find it easier to start rather than stick with a training program. Fifty percent of people drop out of training programs within six months. Once you get past the six-month mark, it is likely that it has become part of your lifestyle and continuing it won't be a problem. The following is a list of common tips that people who exercise as part of their daily lives use to keep themselves motivated.

Training Continuation Tips

- Tailor the intensity, duration, and frequency of training sessions to your level.
- Exercise with a friend.
- Find or make a convenient place to exercise.
- Utilize music that motivates you.
- Set realistic goals.
- Keep an exercise journal.
- Tell others what you are doing.
- Post notes around your living quarters to remind you of your goals.
- Reward yourself for achieving your goals (but not with pizza and ice cream!) with healthy rewards, such as treating yourself to a relaxing afternoon at a spa or a night at the movies with friends.

19

3 THE RIGHT FUEL FOR YOUR BODY

The ability to engage in physical activity—whether the activity is Krav Maga, hitting the weights at the gym, hiking, or just carrying shopping bags to your car—requires a level of good health. In order to perform and feel well in your daily life, you must eat a nutritious diet that supplies the necessary nutrients so that all of your bodily functions are working properly. Every substance that you put into your body has an action or interaction with the cells of your body, so choose carefully.

Fueling the Body

Food is the fuel that your body needs to keep functioning. Just like a car needs gasoline to continue to run. If you were the owner of a Lamborghini Diablo, you probably would not put a low-grade gasoline in it as that might cause the engine to seize up. Think of your body the same way. You must fuel it with a high-quality fuel for it to run efficiently.

Once nutrients are available to your muscles, the muscles are able to utilize energy for muscular contraction. The type of fuel muscles used depends on the physical fitness and workout intensity of an individual. The greater your level of fitness, the more free fatty acids (fat) will be used to supply your body with energy, especially in activities that last more than twenty minutes.

Know Your Nutrients

Nutrients are an important part of a healthy diet and make your bodies perform well. What are nutrients exactly? The components of nutrients are carbohydrates, proteins, lipids (fats), vitamins, minerals, and water. All of these nutrients are necessary for the body to function at all.

Some of these nutrients provide energy, which is needed to generate movement and for workout and exercise. Some of these nutrients are utilized for growth and development of the body as well as regulating the processes that occur in the body, such as digestion, absorption, sweating, and forming new cells.

All Nutrients Are Not Created Equal

You may have heard before that the components of nutrients are not created equal. It's best to choose foods that are nutrient dense, meaning they have many high-quality nutrients Quality is the key word here.

ESSENTIAL

The Food and Drug Administration (FDA) offers a free interactive learning tool to educate consumers on how to read and understand the content of the Nutrition Facts labels that are on all food products sold in the United States. This tool will help you to keep track of calories, as well as provide information that can help you plan a healthy diet. For more information, or to download this learning tool, go to *www. cfsan.fda.gov.*

Most of the foods that are processed and packaged have been stripped of nutrients. Some food manufacturers fortify their products with vitamins and minerals, meaning they add them back into the product after they have been processed out. To fortify a product is better than not having any vitamins at all, but it's not as nutritious or beneficial for your body as nutrients in their natural form. This is why a diet with plenty of fresh fruits and vegetables is so highly recommended. These foods have not been processed and therefore their nutrients have not been stripped away.

22

Carbohydrates

Carbohydrates are a major source of fuel for the body. They are considered sugars and are commonly classified as either simple or complex. Simple sugars are easy for the body to digest, while complex sugars take more time for the body to digest. You will often hear from dietitians and nutrionists that it's important to eat complex carbohydrates because these take longer for the body to break down and utilize and provide a more sustained source or energy. However, the USDA's *Dietary Guidelines for Americans 2005* does away with the simple/complex distinction and recommends fiber-rich foods and whole grains.

Besides the fact that you likely enjoy the taste of carbohydrates, you need sugars in your diet mostly to satisfy the energy needs of the cells in your body. Glucose is the primary source of energy in most cells, and it's produced in your body from the carbohydrates you eat. If your body does not have enough glucose to keep up with the energy demands you are placing upon it, then your body will be forced to make glucose from your muscle proteins. Daily carbohydrate intake should be at least 5 grams per kilogram of your total body weight.

Are Carbs Bad for You?

There are good carbs as well as bad carbs, and you should understand the difference between the two. It's really quite simple. If the food is packaged and or processed, then it's not going to be as nutritious for your body as food that you prepare yourself.

Food that is prepared with ingredients from the earth is going to have nutrients and vitamins that feed your body and are more readily absorbed by it. So try to avoid packaged muffins, cookies, chips, and crackers and try to consume foods that grow in the ground or come from a plant or tree.

ALERT

When it comes to making a healthy food selection, if you are not able to pronounce the ingredients of what you're about to eat, then it probably would not make the list for best possible food choices. Try to avoid processed foods that are loaded with all kinds of additives and preservatives (some of which have even been proven harmful).

If you find yourself in a hurry and need to eat something quickly, which may have to mean something packaged, then there are a couple of things you should look for. Read the list of ingredients printed on the package. Try finding the item that has the fewest ingredients. Next, try to find foods that are made from natural ingredients and that contain fewer preservatives.

Healthy Carb Choices

Good choices for carbohydrates include:

- Brown rice
- Sweet potato
- All fruits
- All vegetables
- Yams
- Whole-wheat pasta

- Brown rice pasta
- Soba noodles
- Beans
- Lentils
- Whole-wheat bread
- Whole-grain bread
- Whole-wheat couscous
- Quinoa

Proteins

Proteins are the main structural material in the body; they are the building blocks of the body. They are a major part of the development of bone, muscle, and other tissues in the body. Proteins are also components in blood, body cells, and immune factors. Although proteins supply some energy, the body uses very little protein to meet daily energy needs.

Most of your protein comes from animal sources such as meat, poultry, and fish. Dairy products can also be considered a source of protein even though they also carry a significant amount of carbohydrates. The source of protein that is commonly overlooked and deserves much more attention is plant-based protein. One of the problems with animal proteins is they usually have high amounts of cholesterol and saturated fats, which can cause plaque to build up on the walls of blood vessels in your body. Plant-based proteins do not contain cholesterol or saturated fats, unless they are added during food processing. This is not to say one should not eat any animal-based proteins. These, however, should be consumed with a level of moderation, and your diet should still include plant-based proteins.

How Much Protein Is Too Much?

In the United States, most of the population consumes about twice as much protein than the human body needs. If you are generally healthy and free from diseases such as hypertension, heart disease, diabetes, and kidney disease, then having extra amounts of protein in your system is generally not going to be harmful to your body. The excess proteins are either excreted or converted by the body into glucose or fat that can be burned for energy.

ALERT

Protein malnutrition can lead to a medical condition known as *kwashiorkor*. Kwashiorkor occurs most commonly in areas of famine, limited food supply, and low levels of education (which can lead to a lack of knowledge on proper dietary habits). An inadequate amount of protein in your body can cause growth failure, loss of muscle mass, decreased immunity, weakening of the heart and respiratory system, and death.

Today, the best estimate for how much protein is required for a healthy adult is 0.8 grams of protein per kilogram of body weight. This amount is higher for athletes, those recovering from illness, and women who are pregnant. Most Americans consume more protein than is recommended simply because they like it and can afford it. Consuming too much protein is usually not harmful to your health.

However, you should know that excessive amounts of proteins are stored by your body in the form of fat or converted into glucose for short-term energy needs. So, too much protein can actually make you more likely to be overweight. Another concern is that high-protein diets can increase the amount of calcium that is lost in your urine. A long-term loss or shortage of calcium in your system can lead to problems with your bone density/ skeletal health and may also be a contributing factor in the formation of kidney stones.

Healthy Sources of Dietary Protein

Some good sources of protein include:

- Lean beef
- Poultry
- Fish
- Beans
- Lentils
- Legumes
- Broccoli
- Low-fat cottage cheese
- Low-fat yogurt
- Eggs

Trimming the Fat

Your body needs very little dietary fat in order to maintain a good level of health. This may be due to the fact that fats and oils are quite dense in potential energy. One gram of fat contains about 9 calories. This is a lot when compared to carbohydrates and proteins, which contain 4 calories per gram.

Although fats are a necessary part of your diet, it is important for you to understand that not all fats are the same. There are two types of fat found in food: saturated and unsaturated fats. Both kinds of fat are found in most foods to some degree. Plant oils tend to have more unsaturated fats while animal fats usually have more saturated fats. Nutritionists recommend dietary choices that have more unsaturated fats than saturated ones. The reason for this is that some unsaturated fats are referred to as "essential" nutrients, or essential fatty acids. These "essential" nutrients are not produced by your body but are needed by it in order for it to perform a number of essential functions. Also, saturated fats have been shown to raise cholesterol levels, which is a major risk factor for heart disease.

FACT

The average American's diet consists of about three times the amount of fat that is needed, and in many cases the fats are derived from saturated rather than unsaturated and essential fats.

Does Fat Make You Fat?

Since the 1980s, food manufacturers have introduced a variety of "fat-free" or "reduced fat" versions of numerous popular food products to the grocery store shelf. Don't let phrases such as "non-fat" or "fat-free" fool you. The important thing to keep in mind is that when the fat is removed from the food, something has to be put in to replace it.

25

Unfortunately, what usually replaces this removed fat is sugar. It is very difficult to reduce both the amount of fat as well as the sugar that is in a food product while maintaining a pleasant taste. For this reason, many low-fat or no-fat products are actually just as high (and sometimes even higher) in calories as regular foods. Most of the time, a fat-free or reduced-fat food product has just as many calories as the original product. Remember, just because a product says "reduced fat" or "fat free" does not mean you can eat more of it without consequence. Most are only fat free until they hit your lips.

ALERT

There is a saying among some nutritionists and dieticians that "a calorie is a calorie is a calorie." What they mean is that removing or reducing the amount of fat in a food product does absolutely no good if the amount of calories is not also reduced. Portion-size reduction is a better method. Think of it this way: Wouldn't you prefer to have just one or two great-tasting cookies than four or five low-fat-and-not-so-awful-that-you-won't-eat-them tasting cookies?

However, when it comes to dairy products, you can safely choose low-fat or reduced-fat products. Milk, cottage cheese, cream cheese, and other dairy products can have reduced fat with very little sugar added. Full-fat dairy products don't taste that much different from their reduced-fat counterparts, so you can cut back the amount of calories by going with a reduced-fat dairy product.

Choosing 2 percent or skim milk over whole milk will cut down on the amount of calories you consume. Of course, dairy fats are derived from animal fat, which can lead to an increase in your body's level of bad cholesterol. An increase in bad cholesterol may put you at a higher risk for heart disease.

Picking Your Fats
Foods with good types of fats include:

- Avocado
- Olive oil
- Canola oil
- Salmon
- Sea bass
- Nuts
- Nut butters
- Tofu

Vitamins and Minerals

Vitamins and minerals are nutrients too. The main function of vitamins is to enable reactions within the body to occur. These reactions help to release energy in carbohydrates, proteins, and fats that can become trapped. This can help all bodily systems, such as digestion, hormone production, and the immune system, work more efficiently. Vitamins do not provide usable energy for the body.

Minerals do not provide energy to the body, but they are critical players in the function of the nervous system, water balance, the skeletal system, and other cellular processes that are constantly occurring throughout the body.

Eating a balanced, healthy diet should give you all the vitamins and minerals your body needs. However, due to the overuse of much of the soil that fruits and vegetables are grown in, most nutritionists recommend taking a multivitamin and mineral that is rich in antioxidants just to be on the safe side.

> **ESSENTIAL**
>
> "Essential" nutrients are nutrients that are not produced by the body but are needed by the body for functions such as the regulation of blood pressure, regeneration of damaged cells, repair and maintenance of vital organs, and cell growth.

Water

Water has a very substantial responsibility within the body. Without water, bodily processes necessary for life would shut down in a matter of days. Water makes up the greatest component of the human body, comprising 50–70 percent of the body's weight. Interestingly, human beings can survive for up to eight weeks without food but only a couple of days without water.

Water has many jobs throughout the body. It acts as a lubricant all over the body—in joints and connective tissues and within organs and vessels—and it even lubricates the body's cells. It also provides electrolytes (sodium, calcium, and magnesium) to the body that are necessary for the balance of fluid compartments found throughout the body.

Water also contributes to temperature regulation, helps remove wastes from the body, and can even act as a shock absorber in some parts of the body.

How Much Water Is Enough?

Adults should drink approximately eight to twelve cups of water per day, maybe more if heavy sweating occurs. If you don't drink enough water your brain will let you know by telling you that you're thirsty. Once you have become thirsty, it usually means you have waited too long to intake water and you may already be dehydrated. It's best to drink water throughout the day to stay properly hydrated.

Fad Diets

Spotting a fad diet is not that hard. All you have to do is ask yourself "Does this sound too good to be true?" If it does, then it probably is. Fad diets often:

- Promote unrealistically quick weight loss (this kind of weight loss primarily results from a loss of body water)
- Limit food selection and have very specific rules, such as having to eat soup for lunch and dinner or drinking their shakes for breakfast and lunch
- Use testimonials from high-profile people or celebrities
- Claim their diet and products work for everyone no matter what age, size, or health problems they may have
- Are often highly expensive

27

Low Carbohydrate or Restricted Carbohydrate Plans

Carbohydrates have been given a bad rap over the past ten years due to fad diets such as the Atkins diet, the Four-Day Wonder diet, and the Scarsdale diet. These diet plans recommend a low or restricted carbohydrate approach to quick weight loss. The primary reason these diets work in the short term is due to calorie restriction. If you eat less than 20 percent of carbohydrates in a day you are most definitely cutting out calories. Carbs are a quick and easy way to eat something that's fast and inexpensive. Think about most snack foods—crackers, pretzels, chips, popcorn—they're all primarily made up of carbs.

> **ALERT**
>
> Eating too much protein, such as the amounts recommended in the so-called low-carb or no-carb diets, requires a lot of calcium from your body. If there is not enough calcium present, then your body may take some from your bones. Maintaining such a diet for an extended period of time, such as several years, puts you at risk for weakened bones due to compromised bone density.

Now take a look at a regular meal. You have a sandwich, a salad, and a soft drink for lunch. The bread from the sandwich is a carb, the salad is all carbs, and the soft drink is also a carb. According to the low-carbohydrate diets, the only thing you are able to eat in that meal is the meat and cheese in your sandwich and a few veggies.

This is merely limiting how much food you intake. This does not seem so bad for one meal, but when you deplete your body of carbohydrates you are depleting your body of energy as well. Without energy it is very hard to exercise, and when you do you are likely to experience a great deal of muscle fatigue and muscle cramping due to lack of proper nutrition.

To Carb or Not to Carb?

Low-carb diets can lead to quick weight loss, but since these diets do not include fruits, vegetables, and whole grains, nutrition experts do not recommend them for a healthy diet. The American Heart Association has also warned against following such a diet due to the high amounts of fats and proteins required for such a plan.

Think of carbohydrates as the fuel for your body. If you are exercising regularly, then you are going to need a certain amount of carbohydrates in order to get through your training session. If you have a day of the week in which you do not have activity, then it may be appropriate for you to consume fewer carbohydrates on that particular day. Think of the car analogy. If you are driving a long distance, you may need to fuel up your tank before you hit the road. Of course, if you are only going to be driving a few blocks and back, there's no need to stop at the gas station.

Low Fat Is Not Low Calorie

Low-fat diet plans usually limit your daily intake of fats to 5–10 percent of your caloric intake per day. The most common low-fat diets are the Pritikin and the Dr. Dean Ornish diet plans. These are not usually harmful to a healthy adult. The problem is they are very hard to stick with. People become bored with the limited choices of food they have. Remember, some fat is needed for the body to function properly. It is recommended to have a little more fat in your diet than the low-fat diet recommends.

ESSENTIAL

You've most likely heard of the Beverly Hills diet or Fit for Life. These diets claim that food gets trapped in your intestinal track and becomes toxic and that these toxins invade your blood and cause disease. This is simply not true. Nonetheless, it has been printed in health-food books since the 1800s. These diets are gimmicks that are designed to sell books.

The Dietary Needs of an Athlete

Athletes need a varying amount of energy depending of their size, body composition, and the type of training being performed. A person who is very small may need 1,500 calories to maintain her body weight, whereas a large person with a great deal of muscle mass may need 4,000 calories to maintain his body weight.

Each individual should start with a rough estimate of what's appropriate for him or her, and calories can be reduced or added from there.

Anyone who exercises vigorously, especially for more than one hour per day on a regular basis, needs to consume moderate to high amounts of carbs. This is considered 50 percent or more of your daily calorie intake. This is why diets like the Zone, which recommends 40 percent of calories coming from carbohydrates, are not ideal for athletes or people who have intense training sessions.

Intake and Activity

Individuals who engage in sixty minutes of exercise per day may need as much as 6 to 10 grams of carbohydrates per kilogram of body weight per day. Athletes who are training for a marathon, triathlon, or those who perform multiple training sessions per day can eat up to 500 grams of carbohydrates per day. They need to consume this amount in order to prevent chronic fatigue and to load the muscles and liver with glycogen (which is the stored form of glucose).

Protein intake for the athlete is 1.2–1.4 grams of protein per kilogram of body weight. It is important that the energy needs are met, meaning the appropriate amount of carbohydrates need to be available. Otherwise, much of this protein will be converted to a fuel source instead of being used for maintaining muscle tissue.

29

Start Out with the Right Diet

For those beginning a strength-training program in which the goal is to put on large amount of muscle tissue, experts may recommend up to 1.7–2 grams of protein per kilogram of body weight. This is up to two and a half times the recommended amount. Keep in mind that the body can only process a certain amount of protein for muscular growth. Any proteins above the amount the body can use to increase muscle protein synthesis will be used for energy needs.

An athlete can eat up to 30 percent of his or her daily intake from fats and oils. These fats should be rich in unsaturated fats and limited in saturated and trans fats.

The vitamin and mineral needs of the athlete are slightly higher than that of a sedentary person. Because athletes eat so much food, they tend to get plenty of vitamins and minerals in their diets. (Unless an athlete is trying to lose weight and is on a restricted calorie diet.) Some experts recommend taking a multivitamin with antioxidants due to the fact that muscle damage is occurring during exercise and many vitamins and minerals can be lost through exertion and heavy sweating.

The Hydration Needs of an Athlete

Athletes, usually experience a great deal of sweating. Sweat is how the body cools itself. If you are dehydrated, your body is trying to sweat and cannot due to a lack of water. This can lead to heat exhaustion and heat cramps can occur.

Heat cramps are muscular cramps that are very painful and last for one to three minutes. Athletes must avoid dehydration at all costs. It is recommended that for every pound lost during exercise due to sweating three cups of water be consumed to replace the fluids.

The Sports Drink Dilemma

Should you drink a sports drink such as Gatorade, Powerade, or All Sport when training? These drinks provide sugar and sodium replacements that are said to increase performance. For exercise that is less than sixty minutes in duration, you should replace the fluid lost from sweat with water. Carbohydrate and electrolyte stores are not usually depleted in this length of time. Anything beyond sixty minutes, carbohydrate and electrolyte replacement does become important and these drinks may be helpful.

ALERT

Many athletes make the mistake of loading up their bodies with sugars before competing, but this is one of the worst things that you could do. Try to avoid sports drinks in the hours preceding an activity. Water consumption is the best method for preactivity or preventative hydration. While sports drinks are often very effective in reducing dehydration, you should drink them during or after hard work or long exercise sessions, but not before.

Marketing protein powders and protein bars to atheletes is another current trend. By eating a variety of foods, such as beans, milk, beef, or fish, throughout the day it is very easy to reach the recommended amount of protein needed per day. Remember, your body can absorb and assimilate only so much protein at one time. When your protein intake exceeds the amount the body needs per day, the excess protein is stored in your body as either fat or sugars. Protein powders can offer as much as 50 grams of protein in one serving. This is half of a 180-pound man's daily needs, without any other food, and most men double the portion size thinking that more protein will make more muscle. If there is any growth in one's physique, it is probably from an increase in body fat rather than an increase in muscle tissue.

Putting It All Together

What does this all come down to? Simply put, it's important that you eat a balanced diet. Each meal should contain a certain amount of carbohydrates, proteins, and fats. Depending on what you do throughout the day and how actively you live your life, the amount of food or calories you need per day will need to be changed to accomodate your specific needs.

Again, think of your body as though it were a car. In order for the all of the parts to work efficiently you need to give it the proper maintenance. A car needs fuel in the tank, oil to lubricate the engine and other parts, air in the tires, fluid in the brakes, and so on. You may be able to drive the car for a while without changing the oil or putting air in the tires, but at some point neglecting its maintenance is going to become problematic.

ESSENTIAL

After you have eaten a meal, you should never feel completely full, "so full you could burst," or as though you have eaten too much. If you feel as though you have eaten too much, then it most likely means that you have. Remember: too much food equals too many calories. Too many calories plus not enough exercise equals unwanted weight gain.

Your body needs high-quality, nutrient-dense foods. A balanced diet consists of three meals per day, breakfast, lunch, and dinner, with maybe two to three small snacks throughout the day. This is not to say that you can never go to a dinner party and enjoy yourself. Just enjoy such things in moderation, not every single night. If you eat well and make good dietary decisions even 80 percent of the time, then there is nothing wrong with splurging the other 20 percent. As long as you are honest with yourself when you are making that rationalization, you should be just fine.

4 THE CARDIORESPIRATORY SYSTEM

Cardiorespiratory exercise is a key component to any training program, especially Krav Maga. Working your body for extended periods of time is impossible unless you've conditioned your heart and lungs to handle the exertion. In this chapter, you will learn to understand how your cardiorespiratory system works as well as how you can benefit from working it. Cardiorespiratory exercise will do more than just help you to improve in Krav Maga; it will also improve the duration, quality, and enjoyment of your whole life.

33

Health, Wellness, and Fitness

These terms are often used interchangeably. Although they all relate to quality of life, they don't necessarily mean the same thing. The definition of health is being free from illness and injury. Notice it doesn't refer to fitness in any way. So it's possible you are in good health (meaning not sick or hurt), but that doesn't necessarily mean you are physically fit.

Physical fitness is sometimes defined as the ability to perform sustained activity without an excessive amount of fatigue. It's very likely that someone who is physically fit has a high degree of good health.

Wellness

Wellness is a popular and more mainstream term for being in good physical and mental health. It includes the physical, emotional, spiritual, environmental, and social aspects of life. Everyone should be concerned with all aspects of health and wellness because they are so closely related to who we are, what we feel, and how we behave. Each one of these components can directly affect the others in a positive or negative way.

For example, if you are having difficulties at work, this can affect whether you're in the mood to meet up with friends after work. The next day you go back to work only to find more difficulties. This drains your energy even more, so you don't feel up to going to the gym. This domino effect is a common obstacle in training. The same is true on the other side of the spectrum.

You may receive a big promotion at work and become enthusiastic in your new position. You become more social, get in touch with your spirituality, and begin training more frequently. The more aware you are of what triggers your moods, the more you will be able to make them work for you instead of against you.

> **ESSENTIAL**
>
> Regular exercise, proper nutrition, and good sleeping habits are all requirements if you are to experience a high quality of health and wellness in your everyday life.

Measuring Your Level of Fitness

There are many ways to measure your level of fitness. The term *fitness* is actually a very broad term. In this case, it's the condition of being physically fit—the ability to perform physical activity in which the heart rate increases and having the ability to sustain that level of intensity for an extended period of time.

With the integration of health, wellness, and fitness into your life it's no doubt that you will look better and feel better. This can be considered a way of living or a way of being that many would term as having a "healthy lifestyle." Individuals who prefer the healthy lifestyle way of living tend to live happy, long, prosperous lives and feel good about their choices in life.

What Is Cardiorespiratory Fitness?

Cardiorespiratory (cardio meaning heart and respiratory meaning lungs) fitness is the ability to utilize large muscle groups for physical activity at a moderate or high intensity or prolonged periods of time. Some may refer to this as cardiovascular (meaning the heart and blood vessels) fitness as well. These terms are often used interchangeably.

The cardiorespiratory system, which includes the heart, the lungs, blood vessels, circulatory system, and the blood, is extremely important. This system must reach every cell in the body. It has to constantly respond to any changes within the body in order to keep all the organs and systems functioning properly. Whether exercising or at rest, this system constantly works to meet the demands of your bodily tissues.

The Basics of Cardio

Activities such as brisk walking, running, cycling, swimming, and cross-country skiing are all associated with cardiorespiratory fitness. Consider for a moment what would happen if you were to go outside and simply begin to run. Consider what the affects of such activity would be on your body.

As you run, your heart rate would begin to speed up; you would realize that your breathing is faster. As you continue to run, your heart beats not just faster but harder, and you may find it harder to breathe. These are normal physiological responses to running. Why does your heart rate increase? Why does your breathing become labored?

Oxygen and Your Body

Whenever you go for a run, your muscles have to contract with more force and at a faster rate than when at rest. The only way your muscles can contract is if they've been provided the necessary oxygen by your blood. No oxygen, no work—it's pretty simple. So where does the oxygen come from?

Not to state the obvious—but this is what your lungs are for. Your heart pumps blood to your lungs, where it picks up oxygen molecules. The heart then pumps that oxygenated blood back out to the rest of your body where it travels through the blood vessels to your working muscle cells. Oxygen is released to those cells, which allows them to continue to contract. The deoxygenated blood is then pumped back to your heart, and the cycle repeats (in fact, this cycle never stops for as long as your heart is still beating). With regular cardiorespiratory (CR) training, the oxygenation process becomes more efficient. As you train, the nine-minute mile you may have run this week will start to feel less difficult three weeks from now.

Benefits and Importance of CR Training

The heart muscle is the most important muscle in your body. You could live without your biceps working, but it's not the same case when it comes to your heart. Many people who work out tend to avoid a consistent cardiorespiratory training program. A regular CR routine has numerous health benefits. In addition to burning calories and decreasing body fat, it strengthens your heart and lungs.

Since heart disease is the leading cause of death in the United States, cardiorespiratory exercise is extremely important and should never be neglected.

Heath Benefits of Cardiorespiratory Exercise

Due to the typical American diet, which consists of large amounts of cholesterol and fried foods, many Americans have been diagnosed with high blood pressure. If you are diagnosed with high blood pressure, you are in a high-risk category for heart disease. Regular cardiorespiratory exercise can decrease your blood pressure almost immediately.

Cardiorespiratory activity also has the ability to speed up your metabolic rate, meaning you utilize more calories with daily activities. This results in a decrease in body fat. The combination of decreased blood pressure and an increase in metabolic rate leads to other health benefits, such as a decrease in resting heart rate, which means your heart doesn't have to work as hard throughout the day. An additional benefit is your body is better able to use oxygen generated energy within the cells of your body, which then leads to an increase in performance in every part of your life. To sum up, the benefits of cardiorespiratory exercise include:

- Decrease in blood pressure
- Decrease in body fat
- Decrease in resting heart rate
- Increase in ability to utilize oxygen
- Increase in performance

Psychological Benefits of Cardiorespiratory Exercise

Psychotherapists, doctors, and exercise experts know that cardiorespiratory exercise has a positive effect on one's psychological well-being. Endorphins, a chemical produced by the body, are released during exercise and communicate with the brain. Endorphins enhance mood, relieve pain, reduce the stress response, and increase the immune system function. Basically, endorphins make you feel good! Other psychological benefits include:

- Decrease in anxiety and stress levels
- Increase in self-esteem
- A renewed sense of value in your personal worth

CR Fitness Tests

There are many ways to test your level of cardiopulmonary fitness. Some of the tests are performed in a laboratory setting. Large pieces of fitness equipment, such as treadmills and stationary bikes, are attached to analytical computers and miscellaneous data recording equipment. The subject is then connected to a great deal of wires and tubes that measure heart rate as well as how much CO_2 is exhaled during the test.

The end result of all of these tests is an accurate record of physiological data from which the evaluators can figure the maximum amount of oxygen that a subject is able to utilize during certain forms of exercise. The greater the amount of oxygen you are able to utilize, the higher your level of physical fitness is going to be.

Here are two tests that you may choose from in order to figure out approximately your own maximum amount of potential oxygen consumption (VO2 max). It's a good idea for you to perform this test before starting any new exercise program. You would also benefit from repeating this test after the first eight weeks of your training. Repeating the test will allow you to compare the figures of your initial test to the new figures, giving you a better all-around picture of the physical results of your training. You may find yourself surprised at the difference in both your ability and appearance after eight weeks of training with a consistent exercise program.

The Rockport 1-Mile Walk Test
Equipment needed:

- Stopwatch (or at least a watch with a second hand)
- 1-mile walking distance (premeasured)
- Calculator (optional)

This test is ideal for those who are unable to run due to injury or from a prolonged duration of no physical exercise. Whatever the case, you should be able to at least walk briskly in order to bring your heart rate up to the 120 beats per minute (bpm) while you walk for one mile. The best place to administer a test like this is on a track. Your local high school or college usually has a track that is open to the public at certain times. Four laps around a standard-sized running track is a total of one mile.

The test requires that you walk as fast as you can (speed walk) for one mile without breaking into a run. Walking is roughly defined in fitness as always having at least one of your feet in contact with the ground at all times. The time it takes you to finish walking this mile needs to be measured and recorded. Immediately after completing your mile-long walk, you should count your heart rate for exactly fifteen seconds. Write down this number and multiply it by four in order to determine your one-minute recovery heart rate in bpm. The equation may appear to be a little messy, but this has been proven to be a quite accurate method.

ALERT

Sometimes high-school jogging tracks are not the standard quarter-mile length. Be sure to confirm the length of the track you will be using in order to prevent inaccuracies in your test.

You may want to fill in your information in the spaces provided below (or make a few copies of this page to use for later tests, such as your eight-week test):

WEIGHT: kilograms (to find your weight in kilos, divide your weight in pounds by 2.2, for example, 120 lbs / 2.2 = approx. 54.5 kilograms)

AGE: years

HEART RATE: bpm (this should be your heart rate at the completion of your mile)

TIME: needs to be measured to the nearest sixtieth (1/60) of a minute (for example, 15:42 = 15.7. Whole minutes are left out. This is figured by taking the seconds and dividing by 60. So in this case, you would divide 42 by 60 to come up with .7) .

VO2 MAX: The formula for finding your VO2 max is gender specific. If you are female, please take note that you should not add the 6.135 below to your total.

$$132.853 - (.1692 \times WT) - (.3877 \times AGE)$$
$$+ (6.135 \text{ for men only}) - (3.2649 \times TIME)$$
$$- (.1565 \times HR) = \text{your VO2 max}$$

For example, if you were a twenty-nine-year-old female weighing 120 pounds with a completion time of 12.6 minutes and a final heart rate of 100 bpm, your formula would look like this: $132.853 - (.1692 \times 54.5 \text{ kg}) - (.3877 \times 29 \text{ yrs}) - (3.2649 \times 12.6 \text{ minutes}) - (.1565 \times 100 \text{bpm}) = 55.60056$ VO2 max. If math is not your strong suit, use a calculator for this.

1.5-Mile Run Test
Equipment needed:

- Stopwatch
- 1.5 mile track, accurately measured
- Calculator

This test is not recommended if you are an unconditioned beginner, have a history of heart disease or heart trouble, or if you've been diagnosed with heart disease or any other heart condition.

In order to complete this test effectively you will need to be able to maintain a jogging pace for a minimum of twenty minutes.

Again, this test should be done on a standard-sized track where one lap will be a quarter mile. You may need to compensate the number of laps you complete if your track is a nonstandard eighth mile or half mile. For a standard-sized track, six laps will be equal to 1.5 miles. If this is the test you choose to perform, it's important for you to evenly pace yourself throughout the test (no breaking into a dead sprint for the last quarter lap). Effective pacing and motivation are key variables to ensure an accurate outcome for this test.

ALERT

There is nothing wrong with pushing yourself to the limit as you near the end of your run or alternating between jogging and sprinting. However, doing either of these during your 1.5-mile run test will cause you to have an inaccurate measurement. Remember to keep an even and steady pace. The point of this test is not to see how fast you can run but to measure your maximum capacity for oxygen consumption.

This test requires you to run or jog the entire distance of 1.5 miles. Immediately after the completion of your run or jog, measure and record the time that it took you. Again, be sure to record your completion time to the nearest sixtieth of a minute. For example, a time of 11:12 will be recorded as 11.2.

This formula is not gender sensitive, so it will be the same for both men and women:

$$3.5 + (483 / TIME) = \text{your VO2 max}$$

VO2 MAX: So if you complete the run in nine minutes, your formula will appear as follows $3.5 + (483 / 9) = 57.16$

Development of CR Fitness

There are a number of methods you can use to increase your level of cardiorespiratory fitness. Any activity that causes your heart rate to increase or in some way places exertion upon your cardiorespiratory system should be considered. Certain movements, drills, or activities are going to cause your heart rate to increase rapidly, while other activities are going to allow your heart rate to increase more slowly and steadily. Both are acceptable methods for cardiorespiratory training.

Activities that allow you to get your heart rate up quickly, such as high-intensity sprinting, are excellent for developing cardiorespiratory strength. On the flip side of this, a moderately paced jog that is performed over an extended duration is excellent for developing your cardiorespiratory endurance. It's important to know the difference between the two and stress both systems in order to be a well-rounded athlete.

Your body will adapt to whatever demands you place on it. When it comes to muscular strength and endurance, the body increases the strength of the connective tissues, and the muscle tissue is able to generate more force (as discussed in Chapter 6).

The result is an increase in strength. When continuously performing any CR exercise, the metabolic system, the pulmonary system, and the cardiovascular system become more efficient.

FACT

If you can't catch your breath, you may need to slow down. As a general rule, a majority of physical trainers claim that you should still be able to carry on a conversation comfortably while working aerobically.

Aerobic Training

Aerobic training is performing any exercise or activity that causes you to become slightly out of breath and that develops your aerobic capacity (*aerobic* means "with air"). When working aerobically, your heart rate is increased above its normal rate and you start to burn fat. However, as you are working you should not be out of breath. You should still be able to carry on a conversation while working aerobically. If you find yourself so winded that you are unable to speak, most trainers will tell you that this also means you are unable to effectively breathe.

Your aerobic capacity determines how efficiently your body delivers oxygen to your muscles and how much oxygen your muscles use for energy. Regular aerobic exercise, such as walking, jogging, swimming, and cycling, increases your body's ability to take in and use oxygen for exercise.

Cardiorespiratory Training and Your Heart Rate

Trainers and exercise experts will tell you that it's necessary to keep your heart rate within a certain training zone in order to burn body fat. The reason for this is that your body will use up more stored fat when you exercise at the lower range of your target heart rate. When you exercise at the higher range, you will burn more calories but it will be mostly in the form of carbohydrates and less total fat.

ESSENTIAL

If you are training for any kind of sport or recreational activity, it's important to train at high levels of intensity for short durations. During most sports, recreational activities, and Krav Maga, your heart rate will reach levels that are very high. Your body should be trained for this kind of physiological demand.

When you work on developing short bursts of higher-intensity activity, your heart rate is going to jump to a higher bpm that is not easy for you to maintain. These bursts cannot be maintained for long, so it will be necessary for you to take a recovery, or an active recovery time, in order to bring your heart rate back to a zone that is both safe and tolerable. This is what is referred to as "interval training."

Sport-Specific Considerations

Think about boxers in the ring. They have to fight two- or three-minute rounds. Within that time period they are going to be working at high-intensity levels where their heart rates are going to be at a high bpm. If boxers don't learn to pace themselves, they will be physically exhausted by the end of the first round. So it's important for boxers to learn not to waste their punches. They move around the ring waiting until they see an opening, then they begin punching and defending. This sudden flurry of activity causes their heart rates to shoot up. They then need to move out of punching range or tie up so they can catch a their breath and bring their heart rates back down before bursting in with yet another flurry of punches when the opportunity is presented. It's for this reason that interval training is absolutely crucial for the regimen of any competitive fighter.

Basketball also shares this need for interval training. Players might be on one side of the court passing the ball, moving left and right and forward and back trying to get the ball through the hoop.

The next moment they may find themselves needing to sprint down to the other end of the court as possession of the ball changes hands. Though this may seem like continuous movement, the heart rates of these players fluctuate a great deal depending on what is occurring at any given moment in the game.

40

Finding Your Zone

The Karvonen formula is the simplest way to figure out where your training zone is. This formula is a mathematical equation developed by researchers that uses your maximum heart rate minus your resting heart rate in order to determine your target heart rate.

Below is an example of the Karvonen formula for a twenty-seven-year-old person with a resting heart rate of 65 bpm:

220 - 27 (age in years) = 193 bpm
193 - 65 (resting heart rate) = 128 bpm
128 x 65% (low end of heart rate) and 85% (high end) = 83 and 109 bpm
83 + 65 (resting heart rate) = 150 bpm
109 + 65 (rhr) = 174 bpm

The target heart rate zone for this person is 150 to 174. So when this person's heart rate is at 150 bpm, he is working at 65 percent of his maximum heart rate. This would be easy to moderate exercise if this person is in decent cardiorespiratory condition. If this individual's heart rate starts to increase to around 170 bpm, 175 bpm, or even higher, then at some point soon he is going to need to take a recovery.

During interval training, athletes try to increase their heart rate up to 85 percent and higher, maintaining this for short periods of time. This cycle is repeated a set number of times or repetitions—three to five times, for example.

Know Your Workout Heart Rate

You can use an electronic heart rate monitor during your own workouts. Many fighters will wear a heart rate monitor on a stationary bike or treadmill. You can still practice interval training, even on a stationary piece of fitness equipment. The electronic monitor will allow you to see and feel how your heart rate fluctuates during training.

You can still employ interval training without the benefit of wearing an electronic heart rate monitor. Whenever you are working your body extra hard you will want to slow down soon after starting to prevent your heart from beating so fast that you are at risk of reaching unsafe bpm levels. If you are struggling for breath, what some call "sucking wind," you've probably already reached 75–90 percent of your max heart rate.

At first glance, 75–90 percent may seem to be somewhat of a wide margin. This range is used because max heart rates differ slightly for each individual. In the exercise world, this is referred to as the *rate of perceived exertion*. You can determine your intensity by how hard you feel you are working. However, be honest with yourself. If you are dishonest, the only person you are going to cheat is yourself.

In Krav Maga there is a great deal of interval training. Intervals are normally performed at the beginning and toward the end of a workout. This ensures that your body has been warmed up enough to prevent any injuries and that you are mentally prepared to work hard. There are three to six different intervals performed during the usual Krav Maga workout. This doesn't mean that you must perform intervals during every single workout you do.

There is something you need to understand about the amount of necessary recovery time between sets of intervals: the more physically fit you become, the shorter the recovery time between each interval.

With practice, you will begin to notice that you are ready for the next interval sooner. As a result, you may want to begin shortening the recovery period you allow yourself between intervals. This will allow you to continually challenge yourself.

Krav Maga Cardiorespiratory Conditioning

Krav Maga fitness emphasizes both cardiorespiratory endurance and cardiorespiratory strength. For the beginning Kravist, it's recommended that you keep your exercises and workout routines at a low to moderate pace. This way you will be able to learn the movements properly, laying a solid foundation from which to build your strength and endurance. This will also help you avoid developing bad habits in technique that can arise from doing too much, too fast, too soon.

ALERT

Interval training is not recommended as a daily workout routine. It's recommended that you take a few days off from interval training every couple of weeks and do only light training and stretching. This will give your entire body the time it needs to properly recover.

Your first few workouts should increase your heart rate and keep it elevated, whether you are using hand weights, punching and kicking the bag, or working on building your core muscles. You may do intervals toward the end of your workout, but it's recommended that you limit them to two or three sets. You're not going to be expected to hold back for very long, only until you've built up the necessary strength in your muscles and joints.

Building on Your Cardiorespiratory Training

Once you've completed three to five workouts, or are at least a few weeks into your workout regimen, your body will have created neurological adaptations to its newly acquired experience of exercise. This means that your nervous system has been stimulated to a point that it has begun to prepare your muscle tissues, tendons, cartilage, and motor skills to be efficient. This means that it's time to pick up the pace!

At this point you may have already begun to notice changes in your body and an improvement in your performance during workouts (even if it's minor). This is when your body's composition begins to change, meaning you will start to see results. Of course, keep in my mind that no two bodies are exactly alike and that this period of time varies from person to person.

You Are What You Eat

For some, change may be rapid and results swift. For others, changes may take a bit more time. Either way, hang in there, keep on going, and you will see results. If your body doesn't change as quickly as you'd like, then perhaps it's time you examine your eating and nutritional habits.

You really are what you eat! If you are not losing body fat and increasing in lean muscle mass, then it's likely time for you to make some alterations in your diet. This doesn't mean you should stop eating! Your body needs food, especially for exercise.

The question is not if you eat but what you eat and how much. For more information on dieting and nutrition, please refer to Chapter 3.

Supplemental Cardiorespiratory Workouts

The following workouts increase your cardiorespiratory strength and endurance and enhance your Krav Maga training. Remember to use the rate of perceived exertion to monitor your intensity level. If you have an electronic heart rate monitor, now is the time to use it. If not, keep track of your fifteen-second heart rate by periodically checking your pulse at your neck.

If you don't have access to a treadmill or stationary bike, you can exercise outdoors, but you'll have to possibly brave occasional inclement weather. In fact, if you prefer riding a bicycle or running on good old-fashioned ground then you should. But maintaining a pace as prescribed below may be difficult without instruments to inform you of your exact pace and the distance you've covered.

Treadmill Workout 1

1. Start with a brisk walk. For most people this will be at a speed of about 3.5–4 miles per hour.
2. Walk for 2–3 minute intervals. Every 2–3 minutes, increase your pace by .2 mph until you reach a point where you feel as though you are working moderately hard.
3. Maintain this moderately difficult pace for an additional 2 minutes. Decrease your pace by .2 (1/5) mph every 2 minutes after that. Continue to do so until your pace returns to a brisk walk.
4. Repeat this cycle 2–3 times. ■

Treadmill Workout 2

1. Begin with a brisk walk for 2–3 minutes.
2. When ready, begin a light jog for another 2–3 minutes (5.0–5.5 mph).
3. Increase the incline to 1.0 and continue jogging for 2–3 minutes.
4. Increase the incline to 2.0 and continue for 2–3 minutes.
5. Increase the incline to 3.0 and continue for 2–3 minutes.
6. Bring the incline back to 1.0 and continue for 2–3 minutes.
7. Repeat this cycle 2–3 times. ■

Stationary cycling (or "spinning," as it's also called) has been a popular fitness trend for several years. Stationary bikes are staples at nearly all modern gyms and fitness/recreation centers. Widespread availability of these machines makes them an excellent supplementary tool for your Krav Maga fitness training. Here are some routines you may want to consider. Remember: Have fun!

Stationary Bicycle Workout 1

1. 3 minutes with resistance at 8 (or equivalent for your machine).
2. 1 minute with resistance at 9 (or equivalent for your machine).
3. 1 minute with resistance at 10 (or equivalent).
4. 1 minute with resistance at 9 (or equivalent).
5. 1 minute with resistance at 8 (or equivalent).
6. Repeat this cycle 3–5 times. ■

Stationary Bicycle Workout 2

1. 3 minutes with resistance at 10 (or equivalent).
2. Keep resistance at 10 (or equivalent) and speed up the legs for 15 seconds.
3. Keep resistance at 10 (or equivalent) and slow down for 15 seconds.
4. Continue alternating your rpms every 15 seconds for a total of 3 minutes.
5. Recover and repeat the cycle at resistance 11 then at 12 (or equivalents). ■

5 DEVELOPING FLEXIBILITY
Bend Before You Break!

Flexibility is an important component in health-related fitness. Lack of flexibility can create functional problems for many individuals. More people are sitting at desks all day, working on computers for long hours, or playing video games, all of which lead to sedentary lifestyles. This behavior can lead to postural imbalances and tight musculature in the neck, shoulders, and back that can become chronic and very painful. This is one of the primary reasons that flexibility training is such an important part of a training regimen.

45

What Is Flexibility?

Flexibility is the ability to move joints through a maximum range of motion without undue strain. Flexibility really depends on the soft tissues (muscle, tendon, ligaments) of a joint rather than the bony structure. However, the structure of the bones in certain joints can place limitations on range of motion. For example, when lifting the leg out to the side, the leg will be able to move into a higher position if the hip is turned out. The reason for this is that the bony structure on the upper leg bone moves out of the way and allows the leg to move more.

ALERT

Overstretching can do significant damage to your joints, especially if you are forcing joints into positions that are not appropriate for you body. When you are stretching it is wise to not force a muscle or joint into a position that does not feel safe. It can damage the connective tissues and cause a great deal of pain.

Strength goes hand-in-hand with flexibility. For the example given above, it's clear that if you turn the hip out before trying to lift the leg, the leg is likely to lift higher. What may not be so evident is that in order to lift the leg there is a certain amount of strength needed to bring up the leg. This is referred to as *functional flexibility*. You have to have the strength to move the limbs through their range of motion, otherwise there is no use for the flexibility.

Importance of Flexibility Training

According to most health professionals, lower back pain is one of the most common complaints in the United States. Poor flexibility in the lower back combined with poor muscle tone in the back and abdominal region is one of the leading causes for this. In addition, lack of flexibility can cause compression of nerves, painful menstrual cycles, and can limit work efficiency.

Because individuals with good flexibility have greater ease of movement, less pain and stiffness in joints, an increase in skill performance, and less chance of injury, it is important to incorporate a flexibility program into your workout routine. In Krav Maga many of the positions involve very large movements in the hips, shoulders, and the spine. Without proper range of motion, the body almost has to fight against itself to perform the Krav Maga techniques well.

Factors Affecting Flexibility

Flexibility is very different from person to person. An individual with very good flexibility in the hips may not have good flexibility in the shoulders. There are many factors that can influence one's flexibility. First is body size, meaning that usually people with high amounts of body fat have a harder time moving their joints through a full range of motion. Usually these people have a sedentary lifestyle so they do not have a significant amount of strength, which as mentioned before is necessary to move body limbs.

In addition, some of the soft tissue on these individuals can get in the way of certain movements, so in certain stretches their bodies have to move more flesh out of the way.

Inactivity and Injuries Affect Flexibility

Activity or inactivity also plays a part in one's flexibility. People who are inactive lose flexibility due to the soft tissues and joints shrinking and losing extensibility. When an individual is not active, the muscles are maintained in a shortened position and more likely to stay that way.

Injury can cause a lack of flexibility. Have you ever had to wear a cast? If one of your joints is placed in a cast, when the cast is removed it is very hard to move the joint that was held immobile. At this point physical therapy is necessary to bring the range of motion back to normal. Similarly, when an injury occurs that does not necessarily need to be immobilized but is painful, the natural response of the body is to avoid movements that hurt. As a result, the area usually becomes tight due to lack of movement.

The Effects of Age and Gender

Age is another factor in flexibility. During early childhood years, kids show an increased aptitude for flexibility. Upon reaching adolescence, however, that aptitude begins to level off. There is a dramatic loss of flexibility with aging, which can be due to failure to maintain an active lifestyle. It can also be related to many of the muscle aches and pains that occur with aging.

Gender can be considered a factor in flexibility as well. In general, females are more flexible than males. It is thought that this is due to a hormonal effect. Males have higher levels of testosterone, which can lead to muscle growth and shortening. On the other end of the spectrum, women have higher levels of estrogen, which promotes muscle lengthening and joint laxity. This is why women who are pregnant become more flexible. The body releases high amounts of estrogen, which allows the joints to become lax. Women need that laxity in order for the pelvis to widen to give birth. This hormone does affect other joints in the body, which is why it's crucial for women who are pregnant (and even after pregnancy) to be careful in how they perform certain stretches.

Experience Counts

Previous athletic experience can also influence one's flexibility. Usually individuals who come from or have experience with sports that require large dynamic movements, such as gymnastics, dance, or martial arts, will have a better range of motion than someone with a sedentary lifestyle. Even a sport you played ten years ago affected learned motor patterns in your body that can benefit you in the future.

Using Your Breath

Controlling your breathing enables you to control other functions of your body, such as heart rate, blood pressure, and respiration. Additionally, conscious deep breathing generates more oxygen for the body and keeps vital lung capacity from decreasing. This can be helpful for cardiovascular activity because it allows more oxygen into the lungs with each breath.

Learning how to breathe can also enhance the mind-body connection. If you are able to connect to your breath you will be able to connect to your higher self. You become more aware of the patterns in your body, both mentally and physically. Next time you are sitting at your desk, stop, take a few deep breaths, and notice what happens to your posture and how you feel afterward. You may notice you sit up taller and feel rejuvenated.

Taking the time to breathe deeply helps to improve your posture and can keep your body from becoming tight and tense. When the body becomes tight and tense, it is very hard to get muscles to lengthen and become more flexible. This is one of the reasons why it is very important to breathe deeply when you are practicing your stretch routine. Through your breath you can stimulate a part of the nervous system that activates the relaxation response. Once you are able to relax you will sleep better, recover from exercise faster, get better from illness faster, and deal with the stresses of life more efficiently.

The best way to use your breath when you are working on a stretch is to inhale as you come up out of the stretch just slightly, then exhale as you move back into the stretch, maybe a little bit further on each sequential breath. Remember: Do not force any stretch. If you use your breath appropriately it will help you relax more into the stretch. Forcing a stretch will make the muscle you are trying to stretch contract and will limit your range of motion. Another way to think of proper breathing is as you inhale you lengthen, as you exhale you deepen the stretch.

Guidelines for Developing Flexibility

There are many different recommendations and ways to increase one's flexibility. Exercise books and videos offer differing advice on what stretch to do, how long to hold a stretch, how often you need to stretch, and so on. The answer to all of these questions is different from person to person and every expert will give different advice. What is important is that you make sure to take the time to lengthen you muscles in some way, whether in a yoga pose, a passive stretch, or some other technique.

Types of Stretches

ACTIVE: This type of stretching is usually used within the warm-up of a training session. You can almost take any stretch and make it active by moving in and out of the stretch using your breath.

DYNAMIC: This is another efficient technique within the warm-up. It involves momentum and muscular effort in order to move primary joints that are going to be used during activity. Big shoulder circles, leg swings, hip circles, and standing spinal rotations are all considered dynamic stretches.

PASSIVE: Within the Krav Maga fitness program, a passive stretch is considered a relaxing, cooling, and calming type of stretch. Passive stretches do not require you to hold your body weight while lengthening a muscle. These are mostly done in the seated or lying down position, and the exhale should be emphasized to recruit the relaxation response.

STATIC: A static stretch is one that has no movement involved but muscles are recruited to hold the position. These exercises are usually, but not always, weight bearing in nature. Holding a High Lunge with your arms over your head, a Downward Facing Dog pose, and a Kneeling Hamstring Stretch are all considered static stretches.

Stretching for Strength

One of the most common questions from a Krav Maga student is how to get more flexible. Flexibility falls under the "use it or lose it" rule. You have to practice consistently, and the one thing people tend to forget is that strength and flexibility go hand in hand.

For example, when trying to bring your leg higher for a kick, most people think, "I can't get my leg up there because I'm not flexible enough." That may be the case, but usually it also involves a lack of strength in the muscles that lift the leg. It goes back to functionality. Your flexibility is only useful to you if you have the strength to move through that range of motion. Both need to be challenged. Static, dynamic, and active stretching have this strength component if done properly. Passive stretching does not involve strength training but is still very healthy for calming and relaxation and should feel really good.

Child's Pose

Child's Pose is a calming position and great for the lower back and hips. From your hands and knees, sit your hips back to your heels and rest your ribs on the inside of you legs. The knees should be apart and the feet should be touching. Your forehead should gently rest on the floor. ▼

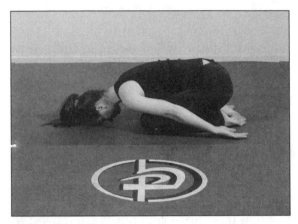

▲ CHILD'S POSE
This is a great position to rest and recover in.

Downward Facing Dog

Downward Facing Dog (or Downward Dog) is a very common yoga pose. It is used a great deal in martial arts as well. The Downward Dog benefits a variety of things in the body. If done well it lengthens the spine and decompresses it from the force of gravity placed upon it all day. It lengthens the entire backside of the body, including the muscles of the lower and upper leg as well as the muscles in the back. Lastly, it strengthens the muscles of the legs and the shoulder girdle.

This position looks like an inverted V. The hands should be shoulder width apart with fingers facing forward, if you feel stiffness in the shoulders, you may want to start with the hands slightly wider then shoulder width and fingers turned out just a bit. The arms should be completely straight, and the muscles in the arms should be active.

The feet should be hip width apart, and if your hamstrings are tight you may step your feet wide and bend the knees as much as needed to move the hips back. This will allow the spine to lengthen and sink both heels closer to the floor.

Don't forget to breathe deeply. This is a great position from which to work on belly breathing, which can help to strengthen the abdominals. It also has energetic effects. When done in longer durations it can lessen fatigue and be highly rejuvenating. ▼

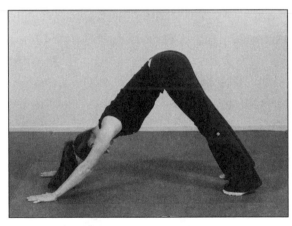

▲ DOWNWARD FACING DOG
Keep your head between your arms and your spine lengthened.

50

Runner's Lunge

The Runner's Lunge position is a very heating position, meaning that you will find when holding it for a long period your body will become warm. This stretch opens the hips and lengthens the hip flexor of the rear leg. If done properly it also can release the lower back and strengthen the muscles of the trunk and lower body.

Place the forward foot directly under the knee, keeping the pressure in the heel of the foot. Try to keep the forward knee at a right angle. The back knee can be either on the floor (Low Lunge) or it can be all the way straight and firm (High Lunge). If you choose to put your back knee on the floor you can add padding under the knee if needed. Remember to keep the integrity of the trunk. Keep the chest broad and the neck relaxed.

Arm placement: The hands start on either side of the forward foot. Once you are stable you may progress the exercise by reaching the arms up overhead. This will challenge your balance skills. Try to keep the ribs compressed onto the wall of the body, which will keep the abdominal wall engaged. Take full, deep, and controlled breaths. ▼

Runner's Lunge with Rotation

With your torso in the upright position, bring your hands to your midline with palms touching. Rotate your torso in the same direction as your forward leg. For example, if your left leg is forward, then your breast bone will turn to the left. This challenges your dynamic balance and wakes up the muscles in the core of your body. ▼

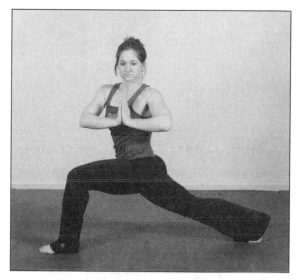

▲ RUNNER'S LUNGE WITH ROTATION
Warms up the lower body and the spine.

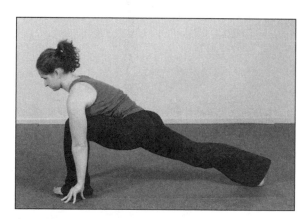

▲ RUNNER'S LUNGE
Avoid letting your knee go farther forward than your toes to prevent knee irritation.

Runner's Lunge with Twist

Place your opposite hand down on floor close to the inside of your ankle. Rotate your torso in the same direction as your forward leg, reaching your top arm up toward the ceiling. With each exhale, see if you can twist a little more. This challenges your balance and lengthens the muscles in your trunk, especially the lower back. ▼

Externally Rotated Runner's Lunge

This position is very similar to the basic Runner's Lunge. The only difference is that both of the hands are placed on the inside of the forward leg's ankle. The forward knee will move in toward the shoulder. Again, the back leg can be on the floor if needed. The external rotation is in the forward leg, so this stretch opens the front hip more than the basic Runner's Lunge. To increase strength, the back leg can be held straight. ▼

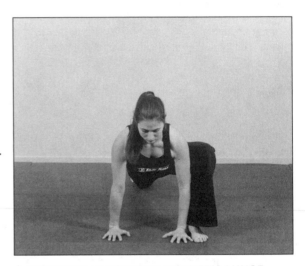

▲ EXTERNALLY ROTATED RUNNER'S LUNGE
Opens the hips of both legs.

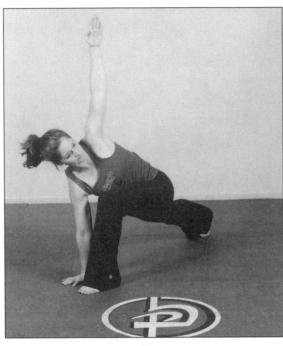

▲ RUNNER'S LUNGE WITH TWIST
Stability and balance are required; remember to breathe.

52

Hamstring Stretch

From a Runner's Lunge position, place the rear leg knee down and extend your front knee all the way to a straight leg. If your hamstrings are tight it is fine to bend your front knee. Place one hand on each side of the body. Again, if this feels challenging, it may benefit you to place blocks under your hands. Try to keep the hips and pelvis square to the wall you are facing, elongate your spine out over your front leg, and breathe. ▼

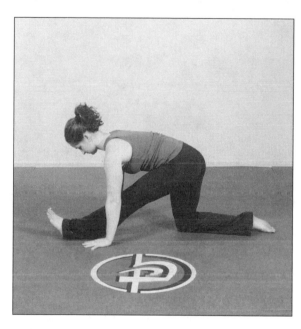

▲ HAMSTRING STRETCH
Good for lengthening the back of the leg.

Cobra

Begin lying face down with your shoelaces facing the floor. Place you hands under your elbows and draw your elbows into your sides. Lift the chest, stretching the breastbone forward and up as you press down into the hands. Look straight ahead and keep your elbows into your sides, relaxing the musculature of your neck. You should feel a small back bend in the upper back rather than the lower back, which is where most people tend to do the back bend. Keep the legs actively reaching back all the way through your toes. This pose increases your range of motion and the lubrication in your spine while waking up the muscles in the back of your body. ▼

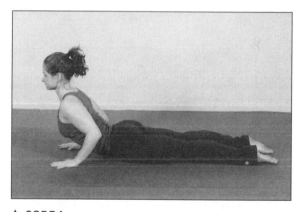

▲ COBRA
This pose may look simple, but it really works the muscles in your back so don't overdo it.

53

Forward Fold

Stand with your feet slightly wider than the width of your hips. Inhale and reach your arms overhead, exhale and take the arms out to the sides. Bend your knees and hinge forward from your hips keeping your spine lengthened. Place your hands on the floor and let the head and neck dangle. Keep your feet parallel to each other and let your body hang over your thighs as much as possible. This is a great way to lengthen the muscles in the back of your body while releasing your neck and shoulders at the same time. Remember to keep your legs firm and upper body loose and dangly.

If you cannot reach the floor, bend your knees or widen the feet. Breathe deeply. ▼

Forward Fold with Wide Stance

Stand with your feet about three feet apart (if this feels too close or too wide, it's fine to adjust your feet for comfort). With a flat back, fold your upper body forward and down so the crown of your head reaches straight down toward the floor. Keep your legs firm and remember to breathe. You can also reach your arms and torso to the right and left side holding for two to five counts. ▼

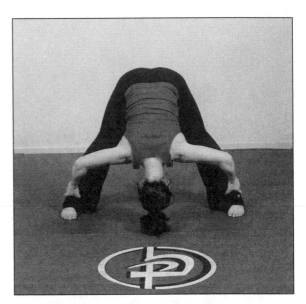

▲ FORWARD FOLD WITH WIDE STANCE
Lengthens the back of the body and inner legs.

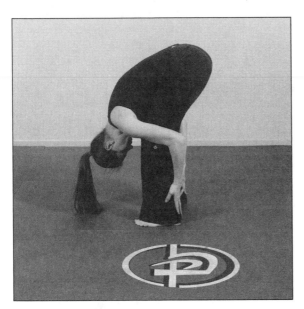

▲ FORWARD FOLD
Lengthen the crown of your head toward the floor to release the neck and upper back.

Happy Baby

Lay on your back with your feet up in the
air and your knees bent. Grab the outside
edges of your feet. Gently pull the thighs
toward the floor as you reach your tailbone
forward. Drop the shoulders down toward
the mat to keep your chest open. Be sure
your head is able to rest on the floor. If you
cannot, place a small pillow or towel under
your head to allow you to rest the neck.
Breathe deeply in order to get a little deeper
into the pose. If you're a flexible person, you
may consider straightening the bottom leg
along the floor. ▼

Seated Straddle

Sit with your legs apart. They do not have to
be as far apart as possible, rather it should
be a comfortable straddle. If you find that
it is hard for you to sit up, you may want to
sit on a blanket, phone book, or something
that elevates you slightly so that you can
sit up tall without struggling to get there.
Start with your arms overhead, take a deep
inhale and rotate your torso to the right, take
another inhale and with the exhale fold your
body forward over your right leg. Try to keep
your breastbone reaching forward toward
your feet to elongate the spine. Repeat on
the other side. ▼

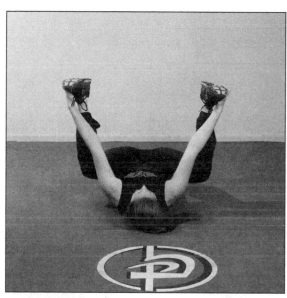

▲ HAPPY BABY
A great stretch for the hips and lower back.

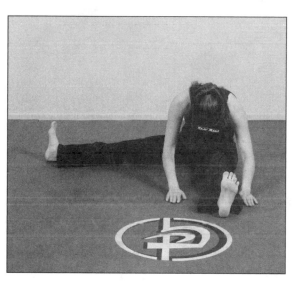

▲ SEATED STRADDLE
Lengthens the muscles of the inner leg.

Seated Lateral Bend

From a Seated Straddle, bend your left knee and bring your left heel in toward you. Inhale as you lift both arms up. As you exhale, take the torso and bend toward the right. The left arm reaches up and over the left ear to elongate the entire left side of the body. Repeat on the other side. ▼

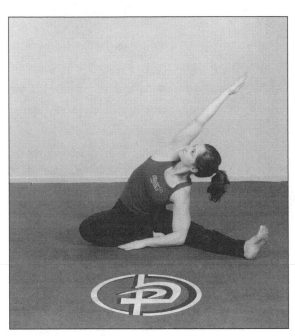

▲ SEATED LATERAL BEND
Lengthens the side of the torso.

Thread the Needle

Lay on your back with your knees bent so the soles of you feet are on the floor. Cross your right ankle over you left thigh. Pick your left foot up off the floor and hold the back of your left leg with both hands. Gently press you right knee away from you as you pull the left leg in toward you. Repeat on the other side. ■

Laying Hamstring Stretch

Start on your back with both knees bent and feet flat on the floor. Use a belt or strap to hold your foot. Wrap the belt around the sole of your foot and extend your leg toward the ceiling. Try to keep the lifted leg straight. ■

Spinal Twist

Lay on your back with your right knee pulled in tight to your chest and the other leg straight along the floor and inhale. As you exhale, drop your knee to the left, reaching your right arm out along the floor, and then look to the right. Take deep breaths and come out of the stretch with an exhale. ▼

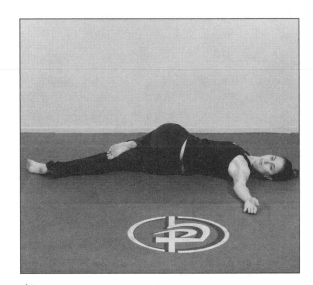

▲ SPINAL TWIST
This is a great stretch for the muscles of the lower back.

Knuckles Behind Back

Reach your hands behind your back, placing your knuckles together. Pull your shoulders and elbows back without letting your front ribs lift up. To progress this, place your hands higher up on the back. This is a great way to open to the front of your shoulders and chest. ▼

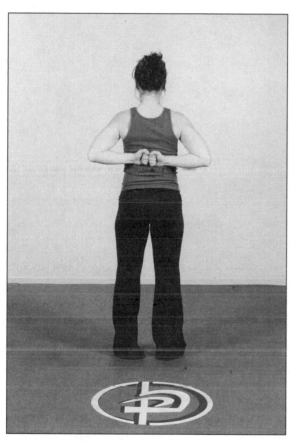

▲ KNUCKLES BEHIND BACK
Expands your chest and opens the front of your shoulders.

Eagle Arms

Hold your arms in front of you, bent at 90 degree angles. One arm reaches under the other as the other arm reaches over. The goal of this position is to try to place your palms into one another. This will take time and practice. In the beginning, your hands may be nowhere near each other. That's fine. Keep practicing and you will get better at this. This is a great stretch for the muscles in the back of your shoulders and in the middle of your shoulder blades, where Krav Maga students tend to experience tightness due to repetitive punching. ▼

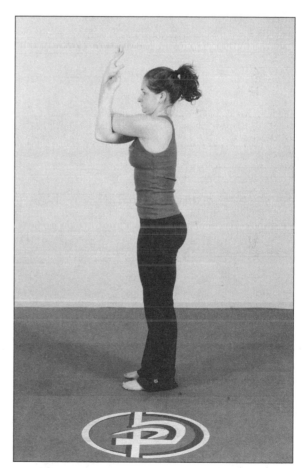

▲ EAGLE ARMS
Opens the shoulder blade region of the back.

57

Flexibility and skeletal mobility are both important elements to any training regimen. The exercises in this chapter, if done properly and regularly, will help reduce your likelihood for suffering the aches, pains, and general injuries that are associated with daily life and physical activity. Flexibility is the key to acquiring a less restricted and painless freedom of motion.

58

6 MUSCULAR STRENGTH AND ENDURANCE

The more you practice punching, the stronger and more defined your arms will become. This increased strength and endurance will allow you to deliver punches faster and for a longer period of time. The more you practice kicking, the better your balance and greater the musculature of your legs will become, allowing you to have more control and stronger knockdown power. Your body's developmental emphasis is placed upon your most recent activities. But don't worry, you can overcome your body's propensity toward inactivity by teaching it new fitness habits.

59

The SAID Principle

The body is an amazing machine. It has a built-in system that makes things easier if you continuously repeat the same movements for a long enough period of time. In the exercise world this is known as the *principle of specificity in training*, or the SAID principle, which stands for Specific Adaptation to Imposed Demands.

The SAID principle refers to the way that the human body adapts to specific types of demands and stresses placed upon it. This is a beneficial function of the human body. In many places of the world this is how people survive. Human beings have the ability to adapt to temperature, altitude, harsh UV rays, allergens, and other environmental stressors. But humans also have the ability to adapt to exercise.

How Your Muscles React to Training Methods

If the body were not able to adapt, you would not be able to increase strength and endurance. For example, if a person consistently lifts heavy weights, that person will develop his strength and muscle mass. If a person consistently lifts lighter weights for longer periods of time, however, then that person will increase his endurance and leaner muscles. When your muscles hypertrophy (increase in size), this is just your body adapting to the demands you are placing upon it.

This principle applies to almost any stressor that is continuously placed upon the body. Have you ever developed a skin callus on your foot? This is the skin adapting to the constant friction placed upon it, say from a shoe for example. If too much friction is placed upon the skin too quickly, what happens? A blister will develop, which is considered a skin injury. This same concept applies within the body. Too much stress too quickly can cause injury. This is why you must progress training appropriately.

Adaptation of the Body to Training

It is necessary for your soft tissues, nervous system, and skeletal structure to adapt to the applied resistance before increasing to higher levels of training. Otherwise, injuries to these areas are more likely to result.

In fighting systems involving kicks to the legs, such as Muay Thai kickboxing, fighters are known to run rolling pins up and down the fronts of their lower legs/shins. They do this in order to strengthen the bone in the lower leg so that it is able to defend against leg kicks with less risk of injury. And yes, according to the SAID principle, it is a good idea for these kickboxers to train their bones to adapt to this kind of serious impact.

Muscular Strength

For many years it was thought that resistance training was inappropriate for many athletes. The belief was that weightlifting exercises would slow athletes down, and the increase in muscle size would cause athletes to loose joint flexibility and become muscle bound. This myth was discarded in the 1960s after coaches and exercise researchers discovered that strength and power training are beneficial for almost all sports and activities.

The formal definition of muscular strength is the ability of a muscle or group of muscles to generate maximal force. The test for finding what your maximum strength is referred to as the one-repetition maximum, or the 1-RM. To determine your 1-RM, select a weight that you know you can lift or press at least once. After a proper warm-up, perform a few repetitions. If you are successful, add some more weight and try again. Repeat this until you are unable to move the weight more than one repetition. The weight you are able to do only one repetition with is considered your 1-RM and is a measurement of your muscular strength. Record this number in a journal, and upon the completion of thirty days of training repeat this test and see how much your strength has improved.

The Need for Muscular Strength

Strength allows your muscle to generate force in short bursts, relying on anaerobic capacity (See Chapter 10 for more on anaerobic exercise.)

Stronger muscles are generally larger and require stronger ligaments (connective tissue) to support them and avoid injuries.

While you can be too flexible, it's hard to imagine a situation where too strong is ever a problem unless your strength is uneven in your body. Each protagonist muscle has an antagonist muscle. Chest muscles overdeveloped relative to the back muscles may exhibit rounded shoulders, shortened pectorals, and otherwise poor posture. While you may want to focus on particular areas, remember that it is essential that you develop your entire body.

Benefits of Strength

As mentioned earlier, muscular strength is essential for a high level of performance in many sports and activities. There are many other health factors that come along with strength training as well. Strong muscles help keep joints strong, making them less susceptible to sprains, strains, and other injuries.

ESSENTIAL

Keeping muscles strong can help make everyday chores and activities much more efficient. When you find yourself on a continuous strength-training program, things like carrying heavy grocery bags, moving heavy furniture, and having to maneuver objects through awkward spaces become easier and less stressful on your body.

Strength training also promotes good posture. Your life is full of activities that pull your shoulders forward, causing a slumping or slouching in the upper back. Working at a computer, driving a car, sitting and reading a book—anything you do that utilizes your arms and hands in front of your body causes gravity to pull you forward and down. This can cause all kinds of neck and back pain, which can then lead to other postural problems and injuries. An adequate strength-training program can eliminate and prevent many of these problems if done properly.

Understanding Muscular Strength

There are two kinds of muscular strength. The first is dynamic strength, or the force generated by a muscle group as a body part is moved. Squats, leg presses, pushups, and bench presses are all considered dynamic strength exercises since movement is occurring.

The second type of muscular strength is static strength, which is built from the force generated against an immovable object. This is also sometimes referred to as isometric strength. Force is generated so the muscle is working, but no actual movement occurs. An example would be pushing against a car. It will take a certain amount of static strength to get the car moving. Once you get the wheels moving, you may start to move your legs. However, your upper body will remain still though it continues to generate force.

Application of Muscular Strength to Krav Maga

Clearly, muscular strength comes into play when you consider any strike, that is, punches and kicks. In Krav Maga you are taught to make every attack count. There is an emphasis placed upon making every attack a strong one. A punch can either irritate or injure depending on the amount of strength you put behind it.

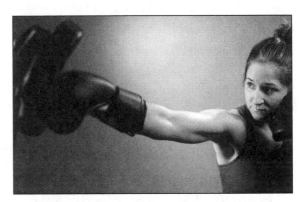

▲ FEMALE THROWING PUNCH
In Krav Maga, you are taught to make every attack count!

Development of Muscular Strength

In general, exercises with so much resistance that you are unable to exceed a minimum of twelve repetitions are the kinds of exercises that build muscular strength. Power lifters, at one extreme, often work with weights that are heavy enough to limit their sets to four or less reps, and they often perform six to ten sets. This type of training effectively develops the greatest potential for maximum strength.

62

Muscular Endurance

Static strength is often associated more with muscular endurance than strength because in order for a contraction to be static or isometric you usually have to hold the position for some amount of time.

When time or duration comes into play, you then need to start working on the level of your muscular endurance. Muscular endurance is the ability of a muscle or group of muscles to make repeated contractions while resisting fatigue. This ability is demonstrated repeatedly throughout your daily life.

The ability to keep going even though you feel completely fatigued is the main goal of endurance. Examples of this could be getting yourself through a long workday then taking your kids to soccer, doing laundry, washing dishes, going grocery shopping, and then ending it all by making sure that dinner is on the table. These are all things that require energy, large movements, and time. On top of that, if you're trying to fit that into one day you are probably moving fast the entire day. This pace can be exhausting and is one of the reasons why endurance training can be beneficial.

Muscular Endurance and the Athlete

If you are a recreational athlete, it is important that you train for muscular endurance. This is due to the fact that your body needs to perform large muscle contractions over and over again in most sports and strenuous physical activities, and especially in Krav Maga. Repetitive punches and kicks require almost every muscle in the body, and the longer your training session, the more endurance you will start to develop.

Development of Muscular Endurance

In order to develop muscular endurance you need to use a moderate amount of weight and resistance and complete sets of slightly higher reps. For example, performing three sets of fifteen pushups will improve your muscular endurance more than doing three sets of five repetitions on a bench press with a significantly heavy load. It's still strength training, but you are creating a longer duration of resistance.

You may experience an increase in your heart rate, which is normal. However, it is important for you to realize that it is not the goal of strength training to get your heart rate up. As you learned in Chapter 4, there is a difference between cardio exercise and muscular endurance training, though the two are definitely linked.

Which Is Better, Strength or Endurance?

Muscular strength and endurance are equally important, so there is no correct answer to this question. It depends on your level of fitness and what your fitness goals are. Strength and endurance can be improved with either program, especially if you understand the relation between the two. Muscular strength and endurance are closely related in that it requires a certain amount of strength to develop endurance. For example, in order to develop upper body muscular endurance through pushups, you must have the strength to do at least one pushup. The inability to do a pushup is a lack of strength, not a lack of endurance.

For the most part, the same exercises are used to increase muscular strength and endurance. The only difference is the amount of resistance and the number of repetitions one completes in a set. In general, muscular strength is best developed by high resistance (heavy weight) and low repetition (short time period) exercises, while muscular endurance is improved by using less resistance (low weight) and higher repetitions (or a longer time period).

Building Endurance Versus Sacrificing Strength

You can have strength without endurance. However, it is nearly impossible to develop muscular endurance without also developing strength. There are weightlifters who can bench press over 500 pounds, as long as they only have to push it up one time.

However, some of these lifters are unable to do twenty pushups. So endurance training supplemented with a weight program is beneficial. While training with low weight may not give you the strength to push up 500 pounds, it will give you the ability to deliver flurries of fast and effective kicks and strikes.

Application of Muscular Endurance to Krav Maga

If you don't knock an opponent out with your first punch, then you'd better have some endurance left to finish the fight. Also, if you don't have the stamina to run away when your options run out or to escape when you see an opportunity, you will have one less option for an exit strategy in a fight.

One way to examine endurance is to consider your ability to convert oxygen into energy and carry away the waste product—lactose. The build up of lactose in the cells is what gives you that burning feeling in your muscles as they begin to fail. Lactose that is not flushed out of the cells during the cool down after your workout is also partly responsible for causing you to wake up sore the next morning.

Having It All

Balancing muscle groups is the key to muscular development. Krav Maga training requires that you develop both strength and endurance because you will need to perform for minutes at a time while maintaining power throughout.

For example, you may wish to break your week up by training for endurance with Krav Maga routines and calisthenics four days a week while lifting weights in the gym on two to three of the days in between. If you want power in your chest muscles, you may want to bench press with 60 percent to 75 percent of your body weight for three sets of five repetitions. For endurance, you would want to lift 25 percent to 50 percent of your body weight for four sets of ten to fifteen repetitions.

If you are new to physical activity but training to get into fighting shape, you should be weight/resistance training at least one to two times per week in addition to your Krav Maga fitness training. You should perform an entire body workout every time you go to the gym. Build up to two sets of ten to twenty reps for each muscle group over the first few months, adding weight each time you exceed twenty reps for a particular exercise.

Next, add sets and lower reps to add strength (at the expense of endurance) for certain muscles while adding reps and perhaps even dropping down to one set for muscles that fatigue too soon (once you are willing to trade strength for endurance).

ALERT

To achieve true fighting shape, it is not recommended that you isolate muscles by days. For example, you should not have a "legs day" or a "bicep day." Every workout should engage your whole body with a series of appropriate exercises.

Within the Krav Maga training system, a combination of muscular strength and endurance exercises are used. These are more commonly known as functional training methods. Following are some functional strength training exercises that increase muscular strength and endurance.

Sumo Squat

This variation of a Squat is easier to learn for many people. It may also be a better choice for people with chronic knee pain. The feet are placed wide and the toes are turned out about 45 degrees. (It's fine if your angle is a little more than 45 degrees.) The torso stays upright as the knees bend over the big and second toes. The hips will not travel back nearly as much for this kind of squat. The pressure is still primarily on the heel of the foot in the upward as well as the downward phase. You may hold a hand weight or a ball to increase the resistance. This exercise is a great way to strengthen, lengthen, as well as open the hips and the inner musculature of the legs. ▼

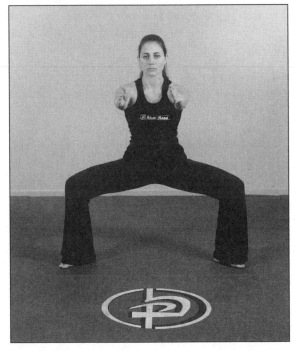

▲ SUMO SQUAT
*Great for lengthening and strengthen-
ing the inner leg musculature.*

The Basic Squat

The squat is one of the most important exercises to maintain a healthy back, hips, and knees. You perform movements very similar to squats all day long without even realizing it. Every time you sit down and stand up you are doing a squat—on and off of the couch, in and out of the car, up and down to use the restroom.

A basic squat is very similar to sitting down and standing up from a chair, which is a great way to begin learning a squat. Find a chair or stool that is close to the height of your knees. Stand with your back to the chair. Place your heels a few inches away from the base of the chair with your feet about a hip width apart or slightly wider. Start with your arms by your sides, and as you take your hips back and down, reach your arms forward to counterbalance your weight. Very lightly touch your hips to the seat and stand back up. Keep the pressure on the heels of your feet in order to make the back of the legs (hamstrings and gluts) do more work then the front of the legs (quads). ▼

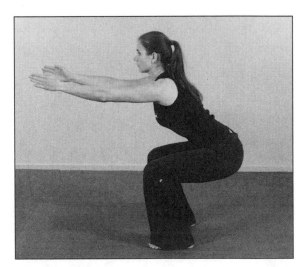

▲ BASIC SQUAT
*Keep the pressure on your heels and elongate the
spine; avoid letting your knees go beyond your toes.*

Squat with Ball

Squatting with a ball works the same muscles in the lower body as a basic squat. The only difference is that you hold a medicine ball in your hands as you squat. (If you don't have a medicine ball, you can use hand weights or even a basketball or soccer ball.) As you drop down into the Squat, touch the ball lightly to the floor. As you come up from your Squat take the ball up over your head, extending through the entire length of your body. Concentrate on controlling both the upward and the downward motions in order to build stability of the exercise. This exercise develops muscular strength in the lower body and the upper body simultaneously. It also emphasizes a great deal of the muscles in the trunk. ▼▶

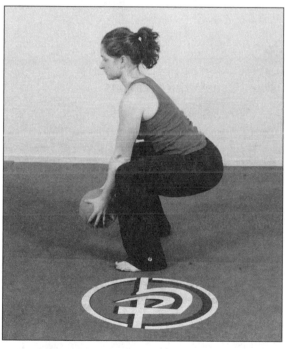

▲ SQUAT WITH BALL #1
Touch the ball lightly to the floor.

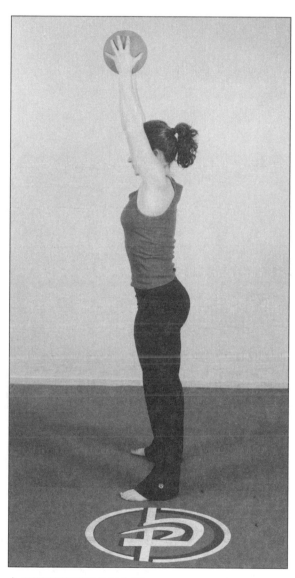

▲ SQUAT WITH BALL #2
Stand and reach straight up toward the ceiling.

Squat with Diagonal Reach

While holding a ball, do a Basic Squat. As you go down in the squat, rotate the torso to the right side, reaching the ball down at a 45-degree angle. As you come up, bring the ball back up diagonally across your body at a 45-degree angle to the left. Be sure to perform the same amount of repetitions on both sides. This exercise builds strength in the lower, middle, and upper body as well as strengthens the ligaments and tendons on the inner and outer knee. ▼

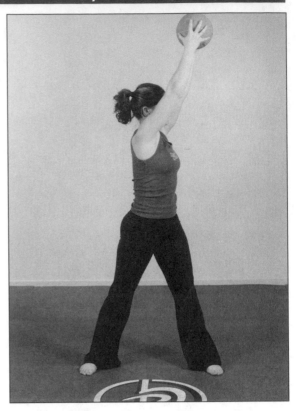

▲ SQUAT WITH DIAGONAL REACH #2
Bring the ball across the body and up at a 45-degree angle.

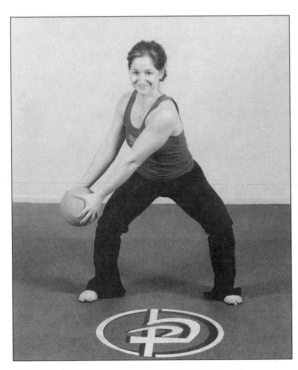

▲ SQUAT WITH DIAGONAL REACH #1
Bring the ball down at a 45-degree angle.

Static Squat with Rotations

You may want to place your feet further apart with the toes turned out slightly for this variation. Come to the bottom of your Squat and hold it. That is the static part. Holding a ball with your arms stretched out in front of you, rotate your torso right and left. Your eyes will follow the direction the ball goes. This builds muscular endurance in the lower body and increases dynamic strength in the trunk. It also develops stability in the inner and outer ligaments and tendons of the knee. ▶

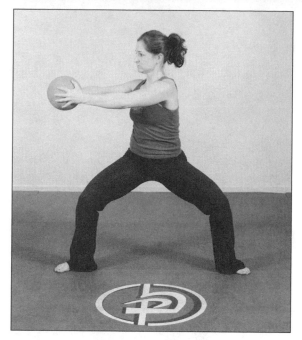

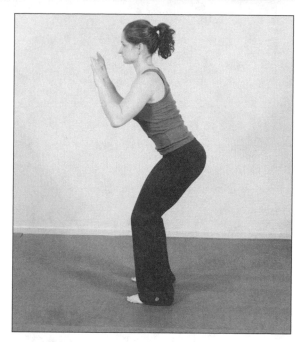

▲ STATIC SQUAT WITH ROTATIONS
Strengthens and stabilizes the knees.

▲ VERTICAL JUMP
Bend the knees and swing the arms down and back.

Vertical Jump

Standing with the feet hip width apart and parallel to each other, bend the knees and swing the arms down and back. As you come up, push off the ground with the legs and swing the arms forward and up. The arms will help to propel the body up and off the ground. Land softly and with control by bending at the knees and hips to absorb the force of the landing. This is an advanced variation of a squatting exercise. It is necessary to build the stability and strength of your squats before moving to exercises that require your body to leave the ground. Exercises that involve leaving the ground are also a great way to develop power. ▶

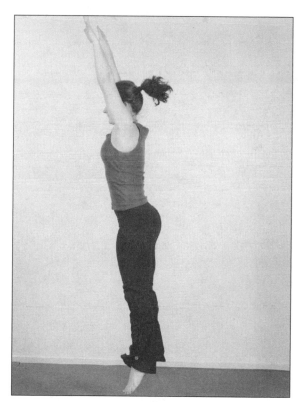

▲ VERTICAL JUMP, CONTINUED
Push off the ground and swing your arms forward and up.

69

The Deck Squat

Begin by standing with your feet hip width apart and arms straight out in front of you. Bend your knees as if you are going to sit on the floor. Once your bottom reaches the floor, roll back toward your shoulders. With momentum, roll forward and place your feet on the floor as close to your hips as posible. Once your feet touch the ground, stand up quickly.

It's fine to use momentum with this exercise as long as you are in control of the movement. This exercise is good for opening up your hips and lower back, as well as for strengthening your knees and hips throughout their full ranges of motion. ▼▶

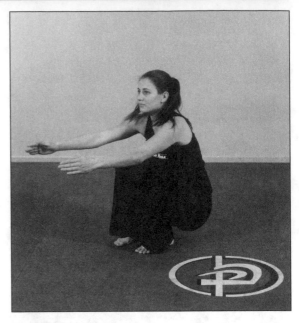

▲ DECK SQUAT #2
Go into a basic squat, and continue lowering your bottom until you are as low as you can go.

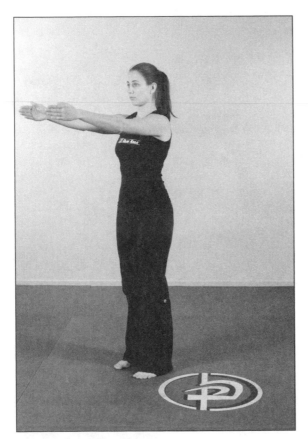

▲ DECK SQUAT #1
Begin standing, feet together, arms straight out in front of you.

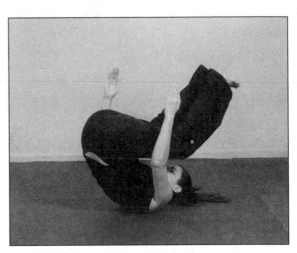

▲ DECK SQUAT #3
Rock back and then roll forward. As you come forward, place your feet as close to your buttocks as possible and lean forward into the squat position. Begin to stand as your feet hit the ground.

70

Stationary Lunge

Stand with feet hip width apart. Step one foot back, placing the ball of the foot on the floor. This is the starting position. Stabilize and balance in this position before moving into the lunge. Bend both knees to about 90 degrees (the back knee will almost touch the floor), then return to the starting position. If you find it hard to stay balanced, use a chair or wall to stabilize yourself throughout the movement. With practice your balance will increase as will your lower body strength. ▼▶

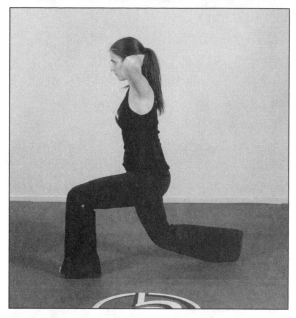

▲ STATIONARY LUNGE, CONTINUED
Bend both knees at about 90 degrees.

Reverse Lunges

Start with the feet hip width apart. Step one foot back and bend both knees into a Lunge. Using mostly the forward leg, pull yourself up to standing. Repeat this exercise with your opposite leg. This exercise builds strength and mobility in the hips as well as increases dynamic balance. ■

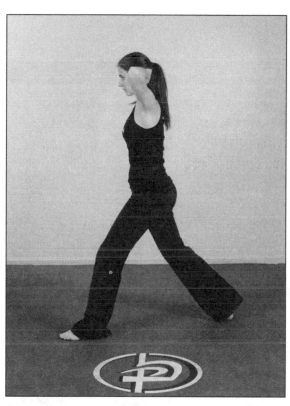

▲ STATIONARY LUNGE
The motion should be straight down and up.

CHAPTER 6   MUSCULAR STRENGTH AND ENDURANCE

Lateral Lunges

Begin with your feet together and arms by your side. Step out to the right, bending the right knee and touching the left hand to the floor. Press off the right leg and bring the feet together. Repeat on the opposite side. Lateral Lunges strengthen the hips and inner and outer ligaments and tendons of the knees. ▼

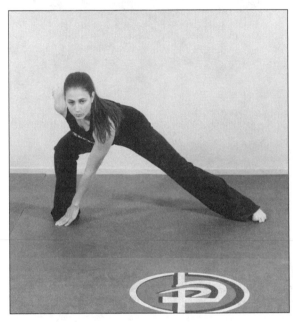

▲LATERAL LUNGE
Lateral Lunge: Step. Touch. Press back to standing.

The Evolution of Your Muscle Training Routine

In order to build a good combination of muscular strength and endurance, you should complete an average of two to three sets with ten to twenty reps per set. Remember that more weight with less reps builds strength, and less weight with more reps builds endurance. You should train for both strength and endurance. Use a weight that leaves you feeling some fatigue by the time you've completed about twelve repetitions. If you complete twenty repetitions with a six-pound ball and you can do another ten reps, it's time to start using a heavier ball!

ALERT

Training injured or damaged muscles is counterproductive. Let your muscles heal before you start working them again. Some muscles recover much faster than others. For example, abdominals, calves, and forearms recover quickly, while recovery of the muscles in your lower back, neck, and hamstrings can take much longer, especially when they have been overworked.

If you are a beginner, start with a ball such as a handball, basketball, or soccer ball before progressing to a weighted ball. When using a weighted ball, the recommended starting weight for women is four pounds and for men at least six to eight pounds. If you do not have a weighted ball, a hand weight will work just as well.

72

7 MUSCULAR POWER

Training for muscular power is a very controversial topic in athletic training. Most sport activities require some sort of powerful movements, so athletes want to be more powerful in order to enhance their athletic performance. But the line between a safe technique or alignment and functionality is often unclear. In order to prevent injuries, training to develop power must be progressed appropriately.

73

The Importance of Developing Power

Because muscular power is not a necessity when performing daily activities, it is not typically considered a component of good health. For this reason, it is not usually emphasized is general physical fitness and wellness programs. Although many of the movements within Krav Maga can be practiced or learned at a slower pace, once the correct motor patterns have been learned, the techniques are then practiced with powerful and explosive bursts.

QUESTION

What is muscular power?
Muscular power is the ability to generate maximum force in the least amount of time. Athletic trainers define it as the ability to release the greatest amount of force in an explosive manner. The equation for mechanical power is: Power = Work / Time. Therefore, if you can keep the same amount of workload, or increase the workload while decreasing the amount of time it takes to perform the work, your power generation will increase.

The development of power is a necessity within a Krav Maga training program for two primary reasons. The first is to make your punches and kicks as effective as possible. Krav Maga would be doing a disservice to civilians if it touts itself as a practical self-defense system but is not effective in reality.

Secondly, power is needed to prevent injury to oneself. Within the Krav Maga curriculum, students are taught to make their attacks with enough power to do damage to an assailant if needed. Knowing how to generate this power is one thing, but having the ability to withstand the power you generate without injuring yourself is the crucial piece of the equation.

Preventing Injury

Training to increase muscular power is important, but it's also important to prevent injury through an appropriate progression in your training. If a new student stands in front of a heavy bag while an instructor directs her to punch the bag as hard and as fast as she can without any other explanation, then it is very likely that this student will end up with an injury to her hand, shoulder, or elsewhere.

A certain amount of training needs to be done in order to make powerful contact to the bag without straining any of the soft tissues. This goes back to the adaptation principle. You need to progress through exercises slowly so that the connective tissues can become familiar with the type of stresses being placed on them. This is why training for power has so much controversy surrounding it. Performing exercises at high forces and velocities significantly increases the risk for injury. But if you are training in a sport that requires explosive movements with large forces placed on the body, the risk for injury increases even further.

So what do you do? You prepare your body appropriately with correct alignment, technique, and awareness so that when you are playing your sport or doing an activity that may be strenuous on the joints, your body has some ability to withstand the forces placed upon it with less chance of injury.

Plyometrics

You may have heard this term used by physical education teachers, athletic trainers, or physical therapists. A plyometric is a type of exercise that lengthens a muscle and then shortens or contracts it rapidly. It usually involves jumping or leaving the ground in some way. Think of it like shooting a rubber band. The further back you pull one end, the farther the band will shoot when released. This is the same concept used when jumping off the ground.

Plyometric drills are a great way to build muscular power in an athlete, but they should be progressed appropriately. The best way to incorporate plyometric training into your exercise program is to first build stability. This means stability in the joint structures as well as stability of the entire body. Balance and coordination fall into this phase as well. Secondly, you must build muscular strength through a large range of motion, for example, full squats and push-ups all the way down and up. This way you have enough strength to support the force that is created when jumping off the ground and to absorb the force when landing back on the ground.

Once stability and strength has been established and achieved it is then safe to add power training through plyometric exercises to your training program.

Stage One: Stability

It is essential that before leaving the ground you are able to or know how to stabilize the joints that are being used to get the job done. This will include the stability of the core, which you can achieve by strengthening the musculature of the core. Be aware that when you are moving rapidly, whether you are leaving the ground or not, you want to have the ability to keep the muscles of the core engaged to support the spine, pelvis, and shoulder girdle. When jumping off using the legs, it's important to be able to stabilize the knee joint.

Individuals that move into a plyometric drill before they are ready usually waggle their knees left and right as they move through the exercise rather than keeping the knee tracking over the big and second toe. This is a knee injury waiting to happen. If you are experiencing this waggle when trying to jump off the ground, do not hesitate to modify the exercise and do either squats, lunges, or some other balance work to learn how to stabilize the knee. For more on drills, please see Chapter 18.

Stage Two: Strength

Once the stability and strength has been set in your ankles, knees, hips, spine, and shoulder girdle it is then time to focus on the muscular strength component.

Since the goal here is to build up toward plyometrics, you should start with resistance training exercises. Once you are comfortable with the movements, you can speed them up as you prepare to take off from the ground. Take a vertical jump for example. You will want to feel as though your squat is solid before adding the takeoff and landing.

Once you have developed a solid squat position with a large range of motion, you can begin to speed up the repetitions of the squat. Control the motion on the way down, then swing the arms up and come up fast by pushing into the ground with your legs. At some point you may just start leaving the ground. Be sure once your feet start leaving the floor that you absorb the landing using your knees and hips. Your landing should not feel jarring on the body at all. If so, go back to the Basic Squat (Chapter 6, page 66) and visualize the downward motion of landing the Vertical Jump 1 (Chapter 6, page 69).

Stage Three: Power Training

Now for the big bang! Power training is very explosive at its highest levels. Plyometrics are a great way to develop muscular power. This can be done with Squat Jumps, Jump Knee-ups, Jumping Lunges, Lateral Jumps, and many other variations.

Plyometrics can be done with the upper body as well. Bursting off of the ground while performing a pushup is one way that you can work your entire body during a plyometric exercise. Using medicine ball drills, such as throwing the ball forward, up, or any other direction explosively, is another way to develop power in the upper body.

Although plyometrics has been discussed as one way to develop muscular power, it's not the only training modality you may use. Any large, strong motion done at high speed is a form of power training. Take a round kick for example. If it's performed slowly, the amount of force used is minimal. It you take the same kick and increase the speed, you are now increasing the amount of power generated behind that kick. And guess what? You did not even have to jump off the ground.

The same holds true for punches and punch-kick combinations. It's simple physics: the force applied to an object equals the mass of what's being applied multiplied by its acceleration (F=ma). So increasing the speed of a kick or punch increases the force. In Krav Maga training, making punches and kicks fast and strong is key. Having power behind the attacks is quite often an emphasis with Krav Maga practitioners.

Squat Jump

This can be done with your feet hip width apart or slightly wider.

1. With your feet about shoulder width apart, sit your hips back and down while keeping your back straight, as if you were about to sit down in a chair, bending your knees in a squat.
2. Place your arms down and back behind you.
3. From the bottom of your squat, swing your arms overhead and push down with your legs, moving your hips forward and up in order to jump off the ground.
4. After leaving the ground you must land appropriately. Use your hips and knees to absorb the landing. You should land back on the ground with a fluid and light movement. The landing should not feel jarring at all. Your arms should swing back upon landing and upward upon the take off. Try to find a smooth rhythm of legwork and arm swing so that one jump leads into the next in a continuous manner.

The faster you are able to generate large forces moving down into the floor, the higher and more powerful your jump will be. Once you are comfortable with this movement you can emphasize jumping higher, or swinging the arms faster, in order to produce more power by using the momentum of the arm swing. The same jump can be performed without using any arm swing at all. Place your hands on your hips and observe the difference in the height of your jump. Without the arm swing this becomes much more challenging. ▶

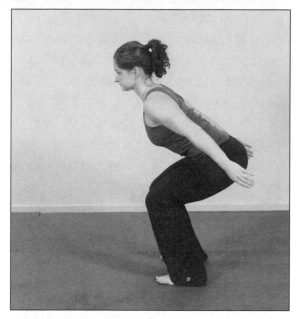

▲ SQUAT JUMP #1
Bend your knees as if you are doing a squat.

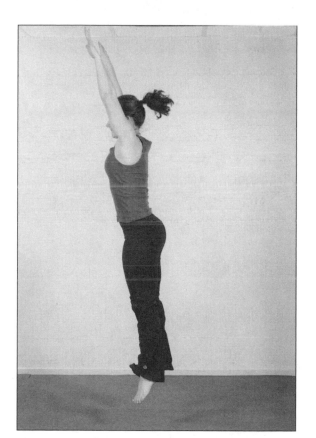

▲ SQUAT JUMP #2
Push down with your legs to jump up off the floor.

77

Platform Jump

Having something in front of you to jump up onto, such as a platform, adds a couple of elements to the exercise. It adds a competitive element either with yourself or with a training partner in that it challenges you to jump higher to get up onto the platform. It also adds a measurable element that makes jumping much more interesting. Maybe your fist platform jump is only eight inches high, but two weeks later you are now jumping onto a platform that is twelve inches high.

1. Stand in front of a platform, bench, or step (between roughly eight and twenty inches high depending on the desired level of difficulty) that has a stable surface.
2. Swing your arms down and back while bending at the knees and hips again similar to a squat.
3. Swing your arms up and burst off the ground, jumping up onto the platform and landing with a light and controlled manner. You may choose to step down in the beginning and repeat the exercise again, or you can jump back to where you started with a smooth and controlled landing.

The progression is to increase the height of the platform as you develop more power. Remember how important the arm swing is for height. If you find you are having trouble jumping up onto a certain height, try using a bigger and faster arm swing. The arm swing tends to be forgotten about when you're focused on jumping onto something that is raised up.

Once you are comfortable with jumping onto the platform, it is time to jump back down. You can do this in two ways. First, jump down while facing forward, again landing in a squat. Once you are comfortable with the height, jump off the platform moving backward, landing in the same spot you took off from. ▼

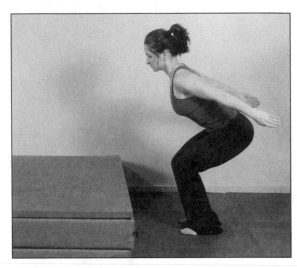

▲ PLATFORM JUMP #1
Bend your knees to prepare for takeoff.

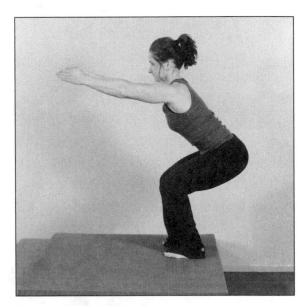

▲ PLATFORM JUMP #2
Jump up onto the platform with a controlled landing.

Horizontal Jump

This jump is more about covering distance than about gaining vertical height. Start this exercise in the same way as you would a Squat Jump. However, the takeoff for a Horizontal Jump should be roughly a 45-degree trajectory that shoots up and to your direct front. This means that the angle of pushoff for your legs is going to be different than it would be if you were jumping straight up.

Again, be sure to control your landing. If you are able to jump so far or so high that you cannot control your landing, then you need to back off on your distance goal until you are able to master a safe and proper landing. You won't be able to improve at this exercise if you injure your legs due to being a little too overzealous in the beginning. ■

High Knee Skip

Think of how you would skip as a child.

1. Swing the left knee up and simultaneously push off the right leg to jump off the floor.
2. The right arm swings forward as the left arm swings back.
3. Land with control on the right leg and step forward, moving right into the other side. Try to continuously alternate right and left with height being the goal rather than distance.

As your knee travels upward, push off the base leg and travel up. Although there is a slight amount of forward travel, the goal here is to go for height. Arm position can be a little tricky with this exercise.

Whatever knee travels upward, the opposite arm swings forward and up. This opposite arm swing is called a cross-extension pattern and is a very functional way to train because it is the pattern humans use to walk or move quickly. Again, be sure to control the landing and try to move from one rep to the next in a smooth and controlled manner. ▼

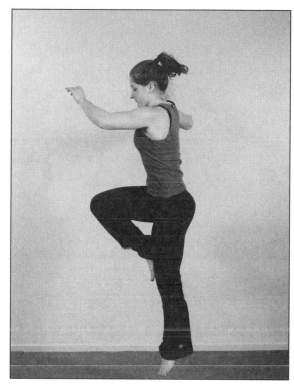

▲ HIGH KNEE SKIP
As your knee comes up, jump off the opposite leg.

Lateral Push

Lateral means to move away from the mid-line. So this exercise is done moving right to left in a continuous fashion. Begin by standing with most of your weight supported on your left leg because this is the leg you will be pushing off from. As your right foot moves to your right, your left leg needs to push off the ground to cover distance. Land on your right leg in control. ▼▶

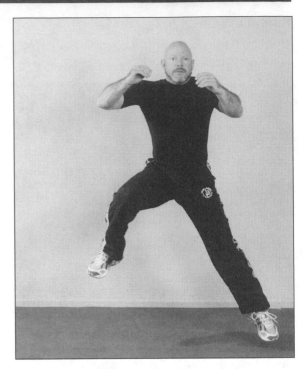

▲ LATERAL PUSH #2
Push off that leg to jump laterally.

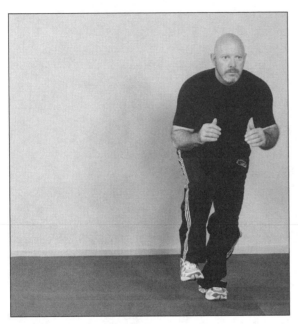

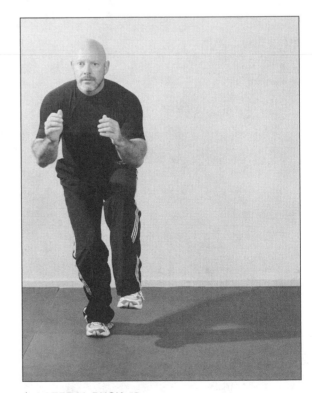

▲ LATERAL PUSH #1
Stabilize on one leg.

▲ LATERAL PUSH #3
Land with control on the opposite leg and repeat on the other side.

80

Remember to absorb the landing by bending at your hips and knees. Keep moving from side to side, each time doing so with a bend and push from your supporting leg. You may find that a slight swing of your arms is helpful in developing a little more power. Your arms will also help stabilize your landing.

SAFETY

The Lateral Push Drill is not meant to develop your speed. So going faster than is necessary or safe is not going to help you improve. Take your time so that you can really develop a nice strong pushoff that can cover an acceptable and challenging distance.

Tuck Jump

This may also be referred to as Jump Knees Up.

1. Bend your knees slightly as you would for a Vertical Jump. Swing your arms down and back behind you.
2. Burst up off the ground while your swing your arms in front of you.
3. At the higest point of your jump, quickly drive your knees up into a tuck position and then release them to prepare for landing.
4. Land softly, absorbing the impact of the landing by bending your knees slightly.

The lower body movement is similar to a Vertical Jump, meaning there is not a lot of knee bend before takeoff. For this exercise, use a large arm swing in order to get enough height to bring the knees up quickly at the top of the jumping phase. ▼

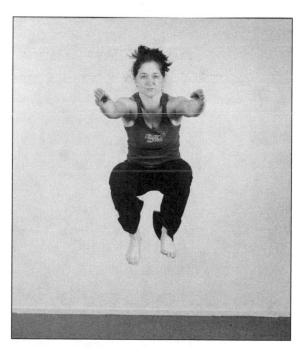

▲ TUCK JUMP
Jump and bring your knees up toward your chest.

81

The Plyometric Step-up

This can be considered a progression to the High Knee Skip.

1. Stand with a step, bench, or platform in front of you. Step your left foot up onto the platform.
2. As you bring your right knee up, jump off your left leg by pressing down into the leg. The arms move in a cross-extension pattern just as in the High Knee Skip.
3. Be sure to come back down with control. The left foot lands on the platform and lowers your weight so the right foot is placed back to the floor.
4. Continue your next rep with the same leg up. As you come down, try not to let too much of your weight shift onto your right leg. To progress this exercise, try to get higher up off the platform with each jump. ▼ ▶

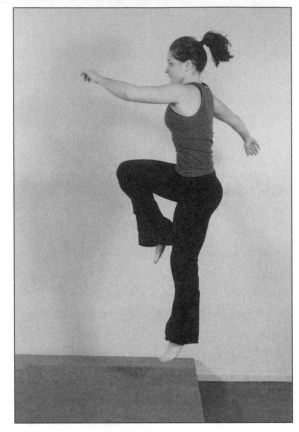

▲ PLYOMETRIC STEP-UP #2
Drive the opposite knee up and jump off the base leg.

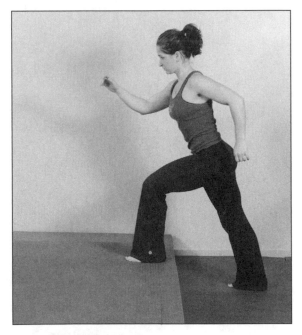

▲ PLYOMETRIC STEP-UP #1
Place first foot on platform.

Jumping Lunges

1. Start with you feet hip width part. Bend your knees slightly and do a small jump, landing at the bottom of a Lunge (Chapter 5, page 52).
2. From the bottom of a Lunge, jump up evenly with both legs, switch your lead leg while in the air, and land in a lunge with your other leg forward.
3. Upon landing, stabilize the lower body then repeat this lunge on the other side. Try to make this exercise fluid when jumping from one Lunge to the next.

You may find it helpful to swing your arms from one lunge to the next. This can also be done without any arm swing to further challenge your leg power. Try making each repetition fluid and controlled, with soft landings from one jump to the next. ▼ ▶

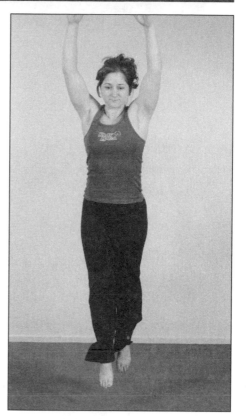

▲ JUMPING LUNGE #2
Jump and switch legs in the air.

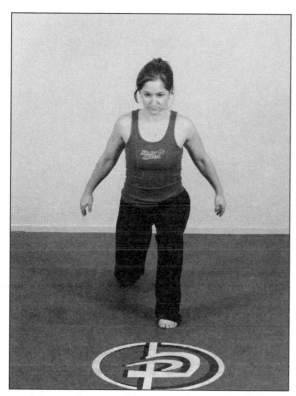

▲ JUMPING LUNGE #1
Start in a lunge.

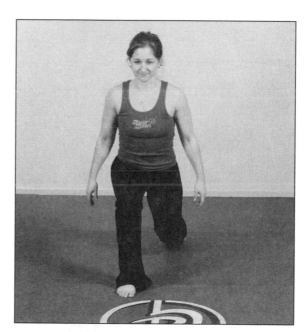

▲ JUMPING LUNGE #3
Land softly with the opposite leg forward.

83

CHAPTER 7   MUSCULAR POWER

Many people relate plyometrics and jumping to the lower body only. In Krav Maga it's important to be explosive with the lower as well as the upper body in order to deliver strong and explosive punches. Training with upper body plyometrics not only increases your explosiveness, it also helps to prevent injury by preparing the body for making contact while punching.

You can also perform this exercise by pushing off the ground and touching your shoulders upon takeoff. Another version is clapping the hands behind the back. One of the most advanced versions is with one hand elevated on a ball and switching hands while in the air. This version is challenging because not only do you have to get more height, but your body has to move in space to switch sides. ▼

Plyometric Pushups

There are a few variations of Plyometric Pushups. Whatever variation you choose, the concept is the same. The first time you perform this exercise keep your knees on the floor. Once you are comfortable and have built some power in the upper body you may do the exercise on your toes. Keep in mind that it is much more challenging for women to do these exercises on their toes. Be smart about your progressions. Many elite female athletes only do these exercises with their knees on the floor.

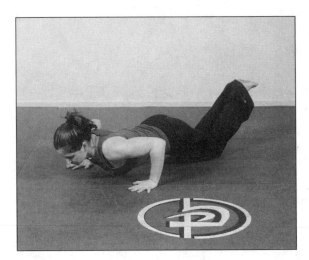

▲ PLYOMETRIC PUSHUP #1
Bottom of a pushup.

1. Place your hands the same way you would for a pushup.
2. Move to the bottom of your pushup.
3. Similar to a Squat Jump, push down with your hands in order to go up.
4. Push with enough force that your hands leave the floor.
5. Clap your hands together (or attempt to do so).
6. Land softly by bending your elbows to bring your chest toward the floor.
7. Prepare for the next rep.
8. Continue moving down and up with controlled landings on the arms.

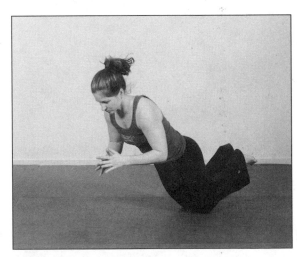

▲ PLYOMETRIC PUSHUP #2
Burst up and clap your hands.

84

When training the muscles of the core or the trunk it's a good idea to train the muscles from both ends. This means that with some exercises you will anchor the lower body and move the upper body, and with other exercises you will anchor the upper body and move the lower body. The following exercises demonstrate each of these types of exercises for strengthening and developing power within the core of your body.

Punch Drill

Punches are covered in depth in Chapter 13, but for the purposes of this drill, here are some tips on delivering straight punches:

- Stand with enough distance from your target to extend your punch all the way—a little more than one arms length from the target.
- Begin in a Fighting Stance (Chapter 13, page 146): face the bag directly; your hands should be at chin height, six to eight inches from the face, with the elbows close to the body to protect the ribs; the feet are shoulder width apart, and if you're right-handed your left foot should be about a step in front of your right foot.
- Keep the elbow down as long as possible as the hand travels forward.
- As you send the punch, the shoulder and hip rotate forward to add power and reach.

- Make contact with the first two knuckles on your punching hand, and rotate the wrist 45 degrees as you make contact.
- Return the hand quickly back on the same path it was delivered on.

Alternate hands while doing two, four, six, then eight straight punches. When the emphasis is on developing power, it is important to remember that you want to keep the strength of your punches while making them faster. The idea is to make each punch fast and strong without losing control of the limbs.

1. Begin in a solid Fighting Stance and start with 2 alternating Straight Punches: a left-right combination.
2. Now perform 4 alternating Straight Punches: left-right-left-right.
3. Move on to 6 alternating Straight Punches: left-right-left-right-left-right.
4. Finish with 8 Straight Punches, leading with the left hand again.
5. Repeat the cycle starting with two Straight Punches. Be aware of your stance and footwork, and generate power from the ground up.

You can also do this drill with a partner who will call out how many punches you are to perform. Another way of doing it is to cycle through the numbers on your own while working your punches to a heavy bag. Keep in mind that it's very difficult to increase the power of your punches without actually making contact. ■

rdddfd _

Kick Drills

Straight kicks are covered in Chapter 14, but here are some tips on delivering straight kicks so you can perform the kick drill:

- Swing the rear leg forward with the knee bent.
- As the hip of the kicking leg comes forward, the knee extends out and recoils back, placing the foot back in its original fighting stance position.
- Make contact with the area of the foot where you would tie your shoes, with your shin, or with the ball of the foot. (In order to make contact with the ball of your foot you need to pull your toes upward to the top of your shoes.)
- You want your foot to travel further than the contact point, so try to kick through the target.

Either alternate your kicks from one leg to the other, or perform the number of kicks all on the same side then switch to the other leg. The idea is that once you begin moving into the kicks you do not stop moving until you have finished the allotted number of kicks.

1. Begin in a solid Fighting Stance and start with 2 alternating Straight Kicks: a left-right combination.
2. Now perform 4 alternating Straight Kicks: left-right-left, right.
3. Move on to 6 alternating Straight Kicks: left-right-left-right-left-right.
4. Finish with 8 Straight Kicks, leading with the left leg again.
5. Repeat the cycle again starting with 2 Straight Kicks. Be aware of your stance and footwork, and generate power from the ground up.

Again, to develop efficient power you have to combine strength and speed with control. One thing to keep in mind when it comes to developing power in your kicks is that you have to make contact to a heavy bag or pad. If you do not have access to a bag, this drill will not work because you cannot put your weight into your kick properly without making contact.

You may take any combination—whether punches by themselves, kicks by themselves, or the combination of punches and kicks—and focus on strength, speed, or power. Focusing on power is the most efficient way for students to understand how to have strong and solid attacks. ■

A medicine ball is a great way to work on strengthening the entire body. It can be a very functional tool because many every-day activities require you to pick things up and move them around in space, which is exactly what you do when training with a weighted ball. You have the ability to move the ball in any plane and any direction, you can throw the ball, and you can hold it for added weight within squats or lunges. It is a very versatile tool and adds some fun to your training sessions.

Medicine Ball Chest Pass

1. Standing firmly on your legs, hold the ball at the height of your chest.
2. Powerfully throw the ball straight out and away from you either at a partner who is ready to catch the ball or at a wall.
3. Have your hands out in front of you, ready to catch the ball as it returns to you. As you catch the ball, bring it in toward your chest to absorb the force in a gradual and fluid manner.
4. Repeat.

Another version of this exercise, which would be considered a progression, is to sit with your feet out in front of you. Place your feet hip width apart and bend your knees at about 90 degrees. Tilt your torso or upper body slightly back to engage your abdominal wall. Holding the ball at your chest, toss it to your partner (who can be sitting the same way) or against a wall. Catch the ball with your hands away from you and bring them in as you catch the ball. ■

Medicine Ball Squat with Overhead Toss

This exercise also has a couple of variations to choose from.

1. While holding the medicine ball at the height of your chin, drop down into a Basic Squat.
2. As you come up, toss the ball straight over your head as high as you can.
3. Catch the ball with your arms extended away from you.
4. Bend your arms to bring the ball back to chin level as you bend into your next Squat.

A slight variation of this is to squat down the same way but throw the ball up high against a wall, absorbing the downward force of the ball as you catch it. Keep your eyes on the ball for the duration of the exercise. ■

Medicine Ball Bounce

This exercise can be done a couple of ways depending on what kind of medicine ball you are using. Not all manufacturers are the same; some balls tend to bounce easier than others, and some don't bounce at all.

1. Make a small jump and at the same time reach the ball over your head then slam it down as your feet land.
2. If you have a large ball that does not bounce well, you may have to get your hands under the ball rather quickly in order to catch it.
3. If you have a ball that does bounce, you can bounce it to a partner, against a wall, or just catch it yourself. ■

Wood Choppers

This exercise, when done correctly, strengthens everything from the legs to all the muscles in the truck to the upper body. It combines lunging, rotating, and reaching.

1. Lunge on the left leg and reach the ball down toward the outside of your left knee.
2. Push off your left leg as you rotate and reach the ball up to the right.
3. Drop back into the left leg lunge and repeat. ■

Other Modalities for Power Training

Olympic lifting has been a commonly used modality to increase power in athletes, including fighters. With Olympic lifting, a large amount of weight is moved in a rapid manner. Lifters must learn to use their legs to generate explosive power. Unfortunately, many of these lifters have a lot of power but zero endurance, as they often have to sacrifice one for the other in order to stay competitive.

You may see individuals performing movements with a weighted bar in which they take it from the floor, toward their shoulders, then over their heads before dropping it back down, this is an Olympic lift. Olympic lifting is a sure way to increase power in any athlete. However, it has its limits. There is not a lot of functionality in the movements you may see Olympic lifters performing.

What Is a Kettle Bell?

The kettle bell is held in the hand and can be lifted, swung, flipped, and thrown. You can move it in an infinite amount of angles and directions, which makes it an interesting and dynamic tool to train with.

One of the primary difference of using a kettle bell rather than a barbell is that the barbell is awkward to bring back down to the floor. This is why Olympic lifters get the weight up and then drop the bar to put it down. Because the slowing down or deceleration process is such a large component in sport, it is crucial to learn how to slow down and redirect the force you are able to create.

Kettle Bell Swing (or Double-arm Swing)

The foundational movement of kettle bell training is what's called a Kettle Bell Swing. It very much like a Vertical Jump and an upper body plyometric combined into one exercise.

1. Begin with your feet hip width apart or slightly wider while holding the kettle bell or weight in front of you with two hands.
2. As you move your hips back down into your squat, the weight will swing back slightly between your legs.
3. As the weight you are using begins to swing forward and up, you must drive your heels and legs down into the floor and burst upward.
4. The weight should propel upward rather than being lifted solely by your shoulder muscles. Think of your hips like an engine and your arms like ropes with hooks on the ends.
5. Power is generated from the ground up through the legs, forcing the bell up and away from you. The bell has to be slowed down with control on the way down and redirected to travel back up again. The same exercise can be performed with one hand at a time as well. ▶

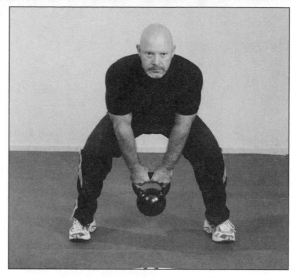

▲ KETTLE BELL SWING #1
Back swing.

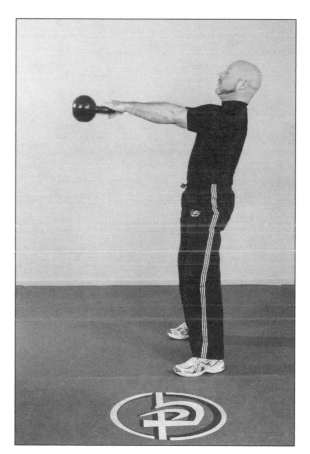

▲ KETTLE BELL SWING #2
Top of swing.

89

8 PROPER WARM-UP AND COOL DOWN

A proper warm-up is a necessity, not only in Krav Maga training but also in any form of physical activity or exercise. Warming up before you engage in strenuous exercise is important for a number of reasons. First, a warm-up reduces your risk of suffering an injury from muscle pulls or strains. Warming up also loosens your joints, gets your blood pumping, raises your body temperature, and increases your overall potential for having a successful workout session before you ever start working hard.

What Is a Warm-up?

Think of your warm-up as a preliminary exercise that's a regular part of your training session. Your warm-up is a crucial part of your workout routine for many reasons. This stage of preparation is meant to prepare your body to meet the demands that are about to be placed on it during your workout or training session.

Coaches, trainers, and athletes, at all levels of competition, preach the importance of a proper warm-up. The need for a warm-up is not restricted to physical (physiological) purposes. Whether or not you warm up before your session can have mental (psychological) ramifications as well.

Physiological Meaning

Physiological refers to what is going on inside of your body whenever you begin to exercise. The term also refers to how the multiple systems of your body are affected by the increase in physical activity.

Your heart and breathing rates will and should increase with any physical activity. Warming up will give your lungs and heart a chance to get moving before more serious exertion is placed upon them. This prepares parts of your physiological system and ensures efficient, safe functions for your heart, blood vessels, lungs, joints, and muscles for the activity that is to follow.

Psychological Meaning

There are also psychological issues to think about as you are warming up. Athletes and competitors at all levels of competition, from recreational to Olympic caliber, often feel that practicing some sort of skill-related activity before competing in an event helps to mentally prepare them. Such mental preparation helps them to perform better at the moment of truth. Whether you are training for a specific athletic event or just getting ready for a jog, mentally preparing yourself to train is essential in achieving a positive state of mind.

Krav Maga movements require accuracy, timing, and precision. These movements require mental concentration and focus. For most Krav Maga students, practicing exercise movements related to the activity that follows has been proven beneficial in improving their skill and coordination for punching, kicking, and putting together striking combinations.

Effects and Benefits of a Proper Warm-up

A proper warm-up increases your cardio-respiratory system's ability to do work. It also makes your body more efficient in the amount of oxygen that it is able to absorb and utilize. This increased efficiency improves the flow of blood to your heart, which reduces your risk of suffering exercise-induced cardiac abnormalities.

ALERT

The amount of time you spend on your warm-up should be based upon the length and intensity of your workout. For example, a fifteen-minute warm-up is sufficient for an hour-long workout at a level of moderate to high intensity. However, a workout of two to four hours in length, within that same intensity range, would need a warm-up of between thirty minutes to an hour.

A proper warm-up causes the body's temperature to rise, thus reducing your risk for experiencing the many exercise-related injuries that can be inflicted upon a "cold" muscle structure. This also protects you from damaging the very precious connective tissue in your muscles and joints. Tendon and cartilage damage can be devastating to anyone, and especially to a competitive athlete.

Increased Blood Flow

Whenever there is an increase of blood flow to the muscles that are going to be exercised, the muscles become warmer and thus more elastic for stretching. Your blood vessels dilate, reducing the resistance of your pulmonary system to blood flow. This decreases the amount of stress that is being put on your heart.

As blood flow increases, the temperature of your blood also increases as it makes its way through your muscles. Hemoglobin more readily releases oxygen at higher temperatures. This translates into an increased volume of oxygen being made available to the muscles you are working, which will improve your level of muscular endurance.

Increased Muscle Contraction Rate

A proper warm-up increases the speed of nerve impulses so that the communication between the brain and the muscles improves, yet another effect of increased temperature and heart rate. An increase in nerve conduction helps your body's ability to move. The increase in your nerve functions will also lead to more speed in muscular transitions between contraction and relaxation.

For example, whenever you deliver a punch, as your triceps contract, your biceps relax. However, when recoiling/returning your punching hand back to its original position, it is now the biceps that contract while the triceps relax. Warming up makes this cycle more efficient and means less energy is wasted.

93

Joint Lubrication

Warming up increases the lubrication of your joints and prepares them for larger, faster, and stronger movements. It is important for your joints to be well lubricated in order to avoid any unnecessary friction. Again, if you begin engaging in strenuous exercise with cold joints, you are just asking for muscular-skeletal injury.

Joint rotations are a critical part of any warm-up, and you should pay special attention to the notorious problem area joints. Professional and recreational athletes alike often experience the same injuries regardless of what sport they play—torn knee ligaments, dislocated shoulders, and displaced hips to name just a few.

Decreased Muscle Soreness

Some researchers continue to debate whether a warm-up will decrease muscle soreness. However, a somewhat general consensus of fitness experts agrees that warming up prior to a workout does in fact decrease muscle soreness if performed during the early stages of an exercise routine.

Another thing to keep in mind is that you may find it hard to get your body moving when you are experiencing muscle soreness as a result of a previous workout. A proper warm-up can help temporarily decrease the amount of soreness you are feeling, making it easier for you to get through future training sessions more comfortably.

You may notice that you feel stiff from not moving. Maybe you sit at a desk at your job all day long or have an unusually long daily commute that has you sitting in a car or train for hours. Getting up, doing a few simple movements, and ending with some light stretching will help alleviate this stiffness as well as cause you to feel energetic and rejuvenated.

Increased Mental Readiness

With a proper warm-up, you may be more likely to go all out in your workout without fearing an injury. Most people have a sense of when their body is properly ready to do an activity. If you do not feel like your body is ready to work harder, kick higher, or punch stronger, it's likely you will not, especially if it feels like it is going to hurt or injure you if you do. This is a perfect example of listening to your body and progressing to the next level of intensity when it feels appropriate.

> **ALERT**
>
> Forget the "no pain, no gain" philosophy when it comes to your body. Pain is your body's most effective form of communicating with you. Listen to what your body is trying to tell you. If it hurts you (there is a big difference between pain and discomfort) to push harder, stretch farther, or kick higher, then don't.

Warming up also prepares your mind to focus sharper on your self as a whole. Being more focused on "you" means an increased awareness of what is going on inside your body. This is important not only to prevent injury but also in helping you to realize when you need to make adjustments in your alignment so you can self-correct any technical points that may be needed to perform well.

General Versus Specific Warm-ups

Warm-ups are usually classified as either general or specific. However, there is a lot of overlap between the two. One type of warm-up is not necessarily better than the other type—they are both of equal importance. Most warm-ups have both general and specific movements throughout.

If you focus too much on either type of warm-up, you will miss out on the benefits of the other. You should try to achieve a balance between both general and specific warm-ups in your routine to achieve a balanced and evenly prepared body that will give you maximum benefits during your Krav Maga routine.

General Warm-up

A general warm-up employs movements that are not necessarily related to the movements and exercises of the workout routine that is about to follow. This type of warm-up includes calisthenics, stretching, and any other kinds of general body movements that make you feel loosened up.

Jumping jacks, squats, lunges, pushups, and sit-ups are all good examples of callisthenic-type warm-up exercises. When performed at a low- to medium-range impact level, these exercises are great to use in a general warm-up. Remember, this is your warm-up not your workout, so don't overdo it. These exercises are meant to prepare your body for your preworkout stretch and workout.

ESSENTIAL

In Krav Maga, you will commonly work on slower movements first before going all out. The same principle applies to your Krav Maga warm-up. This is your time to get your blood pumping and work up a light sweat. Starting out at a high-level intensity or difficulty will completely defeat the entire purpose of doing a warm-up in the first place.

Specific Warm-up

A specific warm-up contains movements that mimic the activity or anticipated movements or exercises that are about to follow your warm-up routine. A specific type of warm-up is a lot like rehearsing a particular skill a few times before doing it at full speed or power.

Baseball players will often swing a bat a few times in order to slowly loosen up their spines, hips, and shoulders. Once they are warmed up, the batters then start to swing a little faster and harder, or may even add some weight to their practice bats.

95

Only then do they step into the batter's cage and swing at a live ball that is being pitched. The same idea holds true for any other sport or physical activity.

Should You Stretch in Your Warm-up?

The first thing that you need to realize about stretching is that it is done during your warm-up routine for far different reasons than when you are stretching to achieve an increase in flexibility. There is a lot of debate and controversy within the fitness community over whether it is necessary to stretch during a warm-up that preceds a training session. There is no one right or wrong answer to this debate as the answer for the individual should be based on a number of factors.

First of all, the need for a preworkout stretch depends on the activity you are engaging in. Krav Maga workouts require very large and dynamic movements with the shoulders, hips, and spine, so it is appropriate to include stretching exercises for these areas of the body as part of the warm-up. On the other hand, if you are going out for a brisk walk, it may not be necessary for you to complete a formal warm-up and an intense prewalk stretch before you step out.

Taking Injury into Account

When warming up, it is important for you to take into account any injuries you may have had. For example, if you recently strained your back, knee, or ankle, you may want to loosen up the affected areas a bit in order to wake up the muscles around the joint.

Please refer to Chapter 5 for more on stretching and strengthening your body safely to avoid injury.

There may be times when you are still healing from a previous injury. In this case, it would be important for you to pay some extra attention to the injured area(s) beforehand in order to warm-up the healing areas more than you normally would. Remember that paying attention does not mean that you should overwork an injured or recovering area or body part. Overstretching or overworking an injured limb will only aggravate the problem further. Finding a balance of comfort and safety is the key. Again, for more information on safe stretching exercises and practices, please refer to Chapter 5.

ALERT

Know your body and listen to what it tells you. If you are stretching your quads or hamstrings, for example, and experience a painful or stinging sensation in your knee(s), this could be your body's way of telling you that you have a torn ligament. Pain is your body's way of telling you to stop. You should not ignore these warning signs.

As you age, you are going to have areas of your body that are more vulnerable to injury or sensitive to movement than others. These areas may also need to be treated with some extra attention and care during warm-ups. For example, if you have an arthritic hip, then that area is going to need to perform some specific warm-up rotations before you are ready to increase the intensity of activity for that area of your body.

Consider the Activity

The next thing that you need to consider is whether the activity you are about to engage in is vigorous, involving large muscle groups. Some exercises shorten and lengthen muscle groups at very high rates, such as running at high speeds or all-out sprinting. If you are going to be running fast or sprinting during your Krav Maga workout, then it would be prudent to perform some hip and leg stretching during your warm-up. Sprinting demands very large hip movements at extremely high velocities and speeds. With this type of movement, you should do some stretching in order to loosen your joints and lengthen the muscles you are going to be using.

In the case of a running or sprinting drill, you would want to stretch your hamstrings, glutes, quads, and calves, as well as the muscles in your shoulders (pumping your arms while running can put a lot of strain on your shoulders). The type of stretching techniques that are recommended for a Krav Maga warm-up are called dynamic or active-static stretching.

These stretching techniques involve large movements and a great deal of muscle fiber recruitment in order to move joints and lengthen muscles to prepare them to work harder. If done appropriately, these stretches will make you feel like you are heating up rather than cooling down, which is considered a passive style of stretching.

Warm-up Guidelines

Your warm-up should be both simple and gradual. It should be sufficient enough to increase your muscle and core temperatures without causing you to experience fatigue or a reduction in your energy stores. This means you should take your time with your first few exercises. By the end of your warm-up you should feel energized and ready to pick up your intensity level rather than feeling as if your warm-up was strenuous enough to be your entire workout. This makes your warm-up highly individualized. A warm-up for an experienced Krav Maga practitioner can completely exhaust someone who is doing Krav Maga training for the very first time. The best way to monitor the level of your warm-up is by paying attention to how your body feels. Your warm-up should be about ten to twenty minutes long to efficiently get the core temperature to increase, lengthen muscles, and lubricate joints. If you are working at too high of an intensity, you will find yourself short of breath and sometimes it can hurt to breathe. If this happens, slow down and focus on taking deep breaths.

97

Considerations of the Krav Maga Warm-up

Due to the fact that Krav Maga fitness requires bursts of high-intensity exercise, there is another consideration that takes on an added significance. Sudden exertion and high-intensity bursts can trigger the onset of myocardial infarction, particularly in individuals who are normally sedentary.

Myocardial infarction is the medical term for a heart attack. As scary as this may sound, for the sake of safety it is important that you understand how your heart and blood vessels are affected by quick bursts of exercise. (To better understand the function of your heart and lungs, along with the effects of heart disease, please refer to Chapter 4 and the section on cardiorespiratory fitness.)

For the unconditioned or weakened heart, the burden of sudden and extreme exertion (caused by genetic heart defects, shock, extreme physical or emotional trauma, or physical activity) may be more than the muscle can bear. Your heart is a muscle and behaves in similar fashion to the rest of the muscles of your body. For example, if you try to bench press more weight than your chest muscles are prepared or able to lift, then those overburdened muscles will give out. This is why weight lifters always use a spotter to help them recover the weight if their muscles fail.

When you are warming up before exercising, it is important to increase you heart rate in a gradual and steady manner. A slow and smooth increase of your heart rate will ensure an optimal blood pressure as well as the proper distribution of blood to the heart muscle.

> **FACT**
>
> Myocardial infarction is a disease of the heart that occurs as a result of an interruption of the blood supply to a part of the heart. The resulting shortage of oxygen can damage and even deaden muscle tissues in your heart.

Unless you are wearing a heart rate monitor, there is no way to determine what your exact heart rate is. In this case you can use what trainers refer to as the rate of perceived exertion. This means that you monitor your intensity by how you are feeling. On a scale of 1–20, with 1 being the easiest and 20 being all-out, 100 percent effort, the warm-up should start at a 3 or 4, increase to 5 or 6 after a few minutes, then increase to 7 or 8 after a few more minutes. The warm-up usually does not go over a 10 on the intensity scale.

Starting Out

Your warm-up should begin with some easy cardiorespiratory exercises. Remember, your warm-up is going to be highly individualized. For a normally sedentary person, this may mean walking briskly for five minutes.

98

Someone with more exercise experience may jog for five minutes. Any exercise that increases the heart rate and respiratory rate will work. Cycling, elliptical machines, stair masters—all are considered cardiorespiratory machines. It is recommended that you perform five to ten minutes of easy to moderate yet continuous cardiorespiratory exercise to begin your warm-up.

> **ESSENTIAL**
>
> Cardiorespiratory exercise—also referred to as aerobic exercise—is a form of exercise that employs continuous, rhythmic activity in order to strengthen your heart and lungs.

Once your cardiorespiratory system begins to work a little harder and your body temperature has increased slightly, you may then begin some dynamic and active-passive stretching. Dynamic stretching involves using movement that takes your joints through their entire ranges of motion. Making large circles with your arms and rotating your hips and spine are dynamic forms of stretching. Even actions that are normally considered physical exercises, such as lunges and squats, can be considered forms of dynamic stretching when they are performed with slow control and held in place instead of completed in steady succession as they are normally done in a workout.

Active-Static Stretching

Active-static stretching is when you hold a stretch from two to fifteen seconds but have other muscles that are contracting in order to assist in the lengthening of the desired muscle. This type of stretch will look very still to the eyes of an observer. However, on the inside of your body there is a lot of work going on to stabilize, lengthen, and create space within your muscle structure. A good active-static stretch will keep the temperature of your body sustained and continue to increase your body temperature depending on the position that you are holding.

People who are generally a little tighter will likely see this type of stretching as very challenging. These people need to keep in mind that it does not matter how far into a stretch you are able to go. The intention of stretching is to lengthen your muscles and move your joints. Again, this is highly individualized and it's important for you to work at your own level.

Proper Warm-up Exercises

Following are some stretches that you may consider using for your general warm-up routine. You can also use the yoga poses for strength stretching in Chapter 5.

99

High Knee Hold

Standing firm on your base leg, lift your opposite knee up and hold the front of your lower leg (shin). Pull your leg in tight toward your chest, holding it for one to two seconds. Release the leg with control and switch sides. This opens up both the hip of your lifted leg as well as the hip flexor of your base leg. ▼

External Rotation Hold

Standing firm on your base leg, lift the opposite knee and rotate it out to your side. Hold the front of your ankle and the heel of your lifted leg. ▼

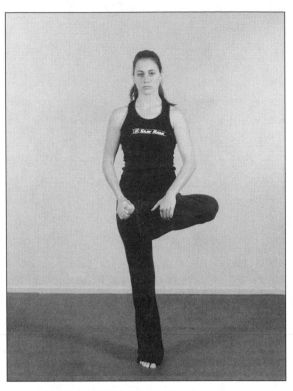

▲ EXTERNAL ROTATION HOLD
Try to stay balanced.

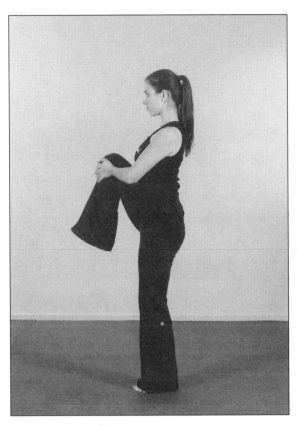

▲ HIGH KNEE HOLD
Lift the knee and hold for two seconds.

Straight Leg Lifts

Standing firm on your base leg, lift your opposite leg up in front of you. You may touch the bottom of your foot with the opposite hand, but this is not necessary. Lower your leg with control and switch sides. This can be done by repeating with the same leg before switching or by alternating back and forth. This exercise lengthens your hamstrings and hip flexors, loosens your hips, and engages the muscles in the trunk of your body. ▼

Standing Quad Stretch

Standing firm on your base leg, reach back and grab the top of your opposite foot, bringing your heel close to your hip. This stretch works on the principle of static balance and lengthens the quadriceps in your bent leg. ▼

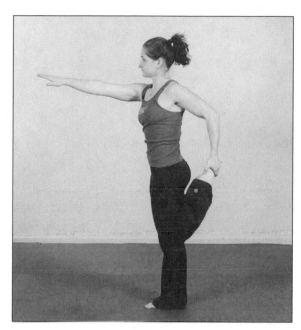

▲ STANDING QUAD STRETCH
Hold for two seconds then release to other side.

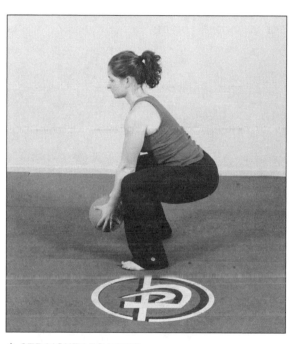

▲ STRAIGHT LEG LIFTS
Lift the leg from the front of the thigh.

CHAPTER 8   PROPER WARM-UP AND COOL DOWN

Standing Quad Stretch with Touch to Floor

This is a progression of the Standing Quad Stretch. Once you have mastered the static balance, try touching the floor with your free hand. This lengthens your base leg's hamstring and challenges your dynamic balance. ▼

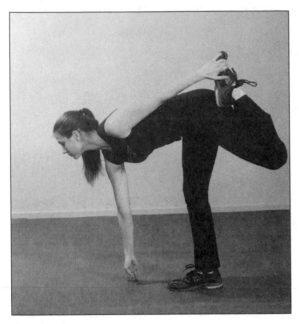

▲ STANDING QUAD STRETCH
WITH TOUCH TO FLOOR
Take your time and stay balanced.

Single-leg Dead Lift

Standing on one leg, reach your opposite leg back and up. As your upper body tips forward, keep your trunk and spine elongated. You may or may not touch the floor then come back to standing. The work is in your base leg, especially the hamstring. ∎

Cool Down

The cool down is the period in which the physiological processes begin to return to their original state. With repetitive motions where muscles are continuously shortening, they may have the tendency to become stiff or feel tight. Within the cool down period, holding static stretches for longer periods is beneficial to bring working muscles back to their original length.

Not only do your physiological processes have to return to their natural states, but your mind needs to come back to its natural state. After your workout, take some deep breaths, relax into some stretches, and observe the effects of your workout. Acknowledge the fact that you are doing something that is good for yourself. Taking the time to be proud of what you accomplish with each workout can make you appreciate it more and keep you coming back for more.

Benefits of Cooling Down

It is thought that stretching to cool down minimizes muscle soreness and is the best time to increase flexibility. Since your muscles are warm and are experiencing an increase in blood flow, it is not uncommon for you to feel as though the stretches you do are becoming much easier.

Take advantage of this time to both relax and enjoy the endorphin rush that often follows a good workout. Use this time to work on your flexibility and to calm your body by taking slow, deep breaths. Move deeper into your stretches. For more information on stretching for flexibility, refer to Chapter 5.

Physiological Effects of Cooling Down

During intense periods of physical exertion, the systems of your body are stressed to their near maximums, leading to an increase in body temperature, heart rate, and blood pressure. In addition, your body also experiences a buildup of biological materials (such as lactic acid) in the muscles. Also, your body releases adrenaline and endorphins into your bloodstream. If you were to simply stop moving after your workout, the levels of adrenaline and endorphins would remain at these high levels, potentially resulting in feelings of restlessness that can cause insomnia later that night. The biological materials in your muscles are known to cause fatigue and stiffness, and a rapid decrease in body temperature, heart rate, and/or blood pressure is extremely unhealthy for anyone.

For these reasons, a cool down routine is beneficial and will help you stay well and healthy in your training. Cooling down allows your body to experience a more gradual decrease in temperature, heart rate, and blood pressure until these finally return to normal resting levels. By gently working the major muscle groups, the biological materials are actively removed from your muscles.

> **ALERT**
>
> During a cool down, your heart rate and blood pressure slowly return to their normal levels. This needs to be done in a gradual manner in order to avoid the pooling of blood in your legs, which can lead to dizziness or fainting. Blacking out can be a real postworkout buzz kill.

As you gently exercise during your cool down, your body will start releasing hormones that will counteract the adrenaline in your system, allowing you to rest and have a good night's sleep afterward. As a result of the increase in the temperature of your body tissues, the postexercise period is the ideal time for you to stretch.

9 BALANCE AND COORDINATION

If you do not practice regularly at finding your center of balance (or challenging your ability to balance), then you will never improve at it. In fact, if you do not practice at it your balance will actually get worse. If a regular schedule of balance training is not maintained, even athletes will begin to find it more difficult to exhibit the high level of grace and stability that is required of them. This chapter explores both balance and coordination and methods you can use to improve them.

What Is Balance?

Balance is the ability to maintain equilibrium against the force of gravity. It is a basic skill needed in everyday life. Your body must constantly make subtle adjustments in order to keep you from tipping over. Try this test: stand with your feet together, arms by your side, and eyes closed. Pay attention to what you feel happening within your body. What you will notice is a constant sway pattern that occurs within the body. This is your body finding equilibrium to stay upright against the gravitational pull toward the ground. Once you close your eyes, balance becomes much more challenging. This is because vision is one of the senses transmitting information to the brain about where and what the body is doing in space.

FACT

Proprioception is the sense of the relative position of neighboring parts of the body. Proprioception is an interoception sense that provides feedback solely on the status of the body internally. It is the sense that indicates whether the body is moving with required effort, as well as where the various parts of the body are located in relation to each other.

Although the inner ear is the balance center, the muscles and joints contribute a great deal to balance as well. The muscles need to have enough strength to support the task at hand, otherwise balance is limited. There are receptors within the joints of the human body that help with balance as well. These receptors send messages to the brain about what the joint is doing (how it is moving and how much force is placed upon it), then the brain sends a message to the muscles to respond appropriately. This is referred to as *proprioception*.

Types of Balance

There are two primary types of balance—static and dynamic. When it comes to balance training, an easy way to understand the different kinds of balance is to examine any of the various forms of dancing. In some styles of dance (ballet, for example), the dancer is required to hold one leg straight out and away from the body while standing on the toes of the opposite foot. Such a position is often required to be held—with little to no shaking, adjustment, or wavering—for a period of time. This is static balance.

You may also see the same dancer execute a high kick with one leg while standing on the other, a movement in which either leg moves up and back down in a strong and rapid manner that can easily throw the dancer off balance, causing him or her to fall. This is dynamic balance. These actions employ two different types of balance, and in order to acquire either, the dancer had to be properly trained. Balance itself is an acquired skill, and such training is necessary in order to develop well-rounded balance skills. However, for most sports and activities (unless they require static balanced positions), dynamic balance is usually considered more functional.

Static Balance

Gymnastics, golf, and tai chi are all excellent examples of athletic activities that require static balance. Static balance is the type of balance that is most commonly thought of when you think of being able to hold your balance well.

This type of balance is exactly what it sounds like—holding a position and not moving. Standing on one leg and holding the other knee up (stork stand) is a static balance exercise.

Static balance training drills in Krav Maga fitness programs are similar to what you would see in most Hatha yoga classes. Standing on one leg with the other leg reaching straight back behind you (Warrior III), or doing the Runner's Lunge while taking your arms up over your head, are excellent exercises that challenges static balance.

Tips for Static Balance

- Begin slowly and take as much time as you need to move into a pose or exercise.

- Take your time and be patient. Every small movement or shift of your body weight changes where your center of mass is within the body, and it takes time for the body to adjust to this.

- While working on static balance, fix your gaze on a single spot. At first it should be about one to two feet in front of you and down on the floor.

- As you become more experienced, challenge yourself by bringing your eyes and chin up little by little. The higher your gaze, the more difficult it is to maintain stable balance.

- It is best to practice static balance poses until you can hold them steady for eight to ten seconds. Do each pose one to two times on each side.

Crescent Pose

The crescent pose is a position that will utilize your legs in very much the same way as the Runner's Lunge or High Lunge (Chapter 5, page 51). Your front leg is going to be bent at the knee 90 degrees while your back leg is extended straight out and back like a kickstand. Next, bring your arms up over your head while keeping your rib cage pressed onto the wall of your body. Try to keep your shoulders away from your ears. Take deep, slow breaths in order to stay calm and focused. ▼

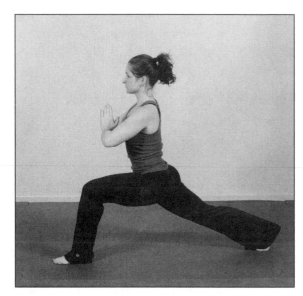

▲ CRESCENT POSE
Bend the front knee 90 degrees and extend the back leg all the way straight.

108

Warrior III

This pose is done standing on one leg with the opposite leg reaching back behind you. Your arms can be alongside your body, out to the sides, or reaching forward with arms by the ears. At first you may bend the standing leg. Once you have found stability, try to make the standing leg all the way straight. The back leg should reach back vigorously with the foot flexed. ▼

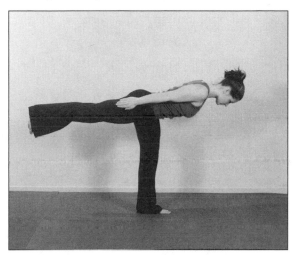

▲ WARRIOR III
Reach back strongly with your back leg and flex your foot.

Single-leg Standing Pose

Begin the single-leg standing pose with the knee of one of your legs lifted up in front of you. Your opposite leg, which is going to be your standing/support leg, should be completely straight. Next, take your bent leg and extend it out in front of you as straight and as high as you can. If your standing leg is bending in order to balance you, then you are not ready to hold your leg so high and you will need to lower your extended leg a bit for the moment. As you improve and become more stable in this pose you will be able to lift the extended leg higher. Avoid lifting your extended leg beyond the point where you can maintain balance while keeping both of your legs straight. Bending your knees is just compensating for a lack of strength or flexibility, so it's more important for you to maintain the alignment then to lift the leg as high as possible. ■

Dynamic Balance

It is an unfortunate reality that training for dynamic balance is often overlooked or overshadowed by static forms of balance training. This neglect of dynamic training is unfortunate primarily because this form of balance is required as much in athletics as in a number of daily activities. Dynamic balance dictates your ability to maintain a level equilibrium while you are in motion. Most martial arts are quite dependent upon dynamic balance. A spin kick, such as you would often see in tae kwon do, can very easily throw the deliverer off balance if that person has not practiced the maneuver enough to maintain balance during its execution. Extending a kick (any kick) out and bringing it back in a continuous manner is just one method of exercise that trains your body for dynamic balance.

Dynamic balance is not only achieved through performing maneuvers with only one support leg, it can also be achieved by practicing and sharpening how you move while in a fighting stance. When in this stance, or working on shadowboxing, you may find that it can be easy to lose control of your balance while learning to shift your weight in so many opposing directions. In this case it is also necessary for you to be able to recover your balance in order to keep yourself moving. The ability to keep your COM over your base of support (in this case your feet) will help to maintain balance while moving.

When performing exercises that train dynamic balance, you should perform eight to twelve repetitions and anywhere from one to three sets of each exercise.

QUESTION

What is a COM?
In any fitness or movement training, COM refers to the center of mass of your body, which is generally located just below the navel and in an inch. The base of support is whatever part of the body is touching the ground. That may be your feet, your hands, or, if you are working on movement on the ground, the side of your body. The center of mass needs to stay over the base of support to maintain balance in any movement.

110

Single-leg Repetition Kicks

While standing on the left leg, bring the right knee forward and up. As the hips move forward, extend the right foot out to complete the kick. Send it out and back in repetition, touching the ball of the foot back on the floor lightly between each kick. Remember, your target is the groin or midsection.

This can also be done with a Round Kick. Turn the base foot out, lift the kicking leg knee up, and extend the kick out and back and again lightly touch the foot to the floor between each kick. Be sure you recoil the kick as this will help you stay balanced. The target for a Round Kick is the rib cage. ∎

Front Kick-Back Kick Combination

Send a left leg Front Kick, place the foot down underneath you, and immediately send a right leg Back Kick. In order to perform a Back Kick, you lift the knee of the kicking leg—in this case it will be the right leg—then extend the leg out behind you. As you kick, think about making contact with the heel of the foot and the toes pointed toward the floor. Recoil the kick and repeat.

The emphasis here is to work on shifting the hips forward and back into each kick. You may look behind you as you send the Back Kick, but it is not necessary for this particular drill. Looking forward and back in repetition can make anyone dizzy, and that's not the best thing for balance. ∎

The Importance of Balance Training

Balance training is actually a great way to prevent injuries. Static balance exercises are a type of muscular endurance activity. What happens is that in order to hold a position (say on one leg for example), all of the muscles in your foot, knee, and hip are activating. They must activate in order to hold you steady. These muscles are usually the stabilizers that do the work.

Anytime you train stabilizing muscles to work you also strengthen connective tissues and joints, and an increase in joint stability and strength equals decreased risk of injury.

ESSENTIAL

Human beings lose most of their natural balance after age twenty-five. This is part of the reason that elderly people can fall so easily. If they do not practice maintaining balance, they can easily lose balance, possibly leading to a fall that could result in a serious injury.

The body is always looking to find a state of equilibrium. As you age, this process that is controlled by the nervous system begins to slow down. This slowing down process is inevitable, but with training you can prolong the process and live life to the fullest whatever your age.

111

Practicing balance exercises challenges the nervous system and helps keep the mind-body connection sharp. It also helps to keep the mind and body sharp in the case that balance has to be regained. It has happened to us all at some point—tripping over a parking block or missing that last step. Without any balance practice your response to regaining balance is slow. In the instance that you may be falling, it is crucial to be able to regain balance quickly.

In a martial arts or self-defense setting, you may find that you get pushed or shoved by someone who may be a threat or someone your may be training with. It's important that you are able to regain your balance in these situations. Similarly, if you send a kick that was not as accurate as you thought it was going to be, you may find that you need to find your center and realign your body before continuing on to the next movement.

Coordination

How your brain and body organizes muscle contractions so that a skill or task can be accomplished is called coordination. Coordination is an interesting and complex concept. When you are learning or doing exercises that involve moving your body or body parts in many directions repetitively, the connection between the brain and the body can become confused.

This is when people will usually say, "I'm not coordinated enough for this!" Once most people get to the point where they cannot keep up with the movements, it is usually too much for their brain and body to coordinate and they become frustrated. Does that mean you can't do it at all? Absolutely not! You have to find a way to make the skills make sense to your body before you progress to the next level of complexity.

> **QUESTION**
>
> **How do you develop better coordination?**
> Coordination will improve with practice and appropriate progressions. Remember the saying "practice makes perfect"? This has some truth to it. Keep in mind that it is important to practice at your skill level before advancing to the next level in order to build a solid foundation to progress from. It may be more beneficial to say "perfect practice makes perfect."

If a student is not given enough time to properly and gradually progress in coordination and balance training, the result would likely be disastrous. The student's arms will likely flail all over the place, his weight would move in the wrong direction, and his feet would move incorrectly. The correct way to teach these elements to a student so that he does not become overly frustrated would be to teach only a combination of simplistic movements (four straight punches, for example) in the beginning. This helps beginning students avoid thinking that they are too uncoordinated for Krav Maga.

Beginner students must master these initial four straight punches before moving on. Once they have, the instructor can then move on to teach them hook punches, then uppercuts, and so on. Once they've reached this point, it may be appropriate to integrate three or four different punches into a short punching combination. More often than not, the average beginner (depending on previous experience) takes at least one year of training in order to master that first particular combination alone with any quality. Of course, this amount of time could be shorter or longer for you depending on how much time, sweat, and effort you are willing to put into it.

Types of Coordination

There are several types of coordination. The first type is coordinating left and right. Combinations and sequencing of exercises can get confusing at first when you constantly have to think about left and right sides having a job to do. It's best to learn the movements on one side and then switch sides. This goes for punch combination as well as for something like lunges.

Coordinating your top and bottom, the second type of coordination, relates to exercises that require you to focus on your upper body while your lower body is doing something else at the same time. All Krav Maga movements require you to do this, at least to some extent. In the beginning stages of your Krav Maga training, these two halves of your body may not come together with the correct timing. With time and regular practice, you will improve and your movements will begin to occur naturally in a more efficient and coordinated manner.

Improving Coordination

For someone who is very new to the mechanics of punching, a left Straight Punch-right Straight Punch-left Hook-right Uppercut combination may be a bit too complex to put together in a smooth, fluid manner.

This is due to the fact that this combination requires you to transition your momentum from one direction to another rather quickly—first forward with your Straight Punches, shifting to the side to deliver your Hook Punch, then pulling up the shoulders to throw your Uppercut. To accomplish all those punches, you have to alternate your legs and hips from left to right the entire time.

ALERT

Don't be alarmed! You will coordinate left and right with the top and bottom without having to think about it too much. Being in tune with your breathing is very helpful. It's kind of like playing the drums. The feet and hands are doing two separate things. With practice, all limbs will become coordinated in the correct manner and will work together nicely.

It will take time and a lot of practice in order for you to break down these skills into separate components in such a way that will allow your brain a chance to absorb and organize the variety of complex movements. If your body was a car, your brain would be the steering wheel, accelerator, brake, and turn signals all rolled into one. Your brain must first grasp the techniques and combinations before your body can perform them well.

CHAPTER 9 BALANCE AND COORDINATION

10 FIT TO FIGHT

Why is Krav Maga such an effective form of fitness? The act of fighting is one of the most physically taxing activities on the planet. When you punch, you extend your weight outwards, putting as much force behind your fist as possible. Why? Because when you land a punch, you want it to do as much damage as possible. However, it takes far more force to miss than it does to land a punch. What does this mean for you? This means that if your first punch (or even the first few) does not land, you are going to need to have the stamina to go the distance. And in order to do that, you will need to be fit enough to fight.

Be Prepared

At some point (the sooner the better), you will want to get a heart rate monitor. A heart monitor is essential if you want to accurately manage your efforts to achieve certain goals or manage the balance between aerobic and anaerobic conditioning, fat loss, or cardio threshold conditioning. Only with a heart monitor can you know for sure that you have worked out at an intensity level appropriate to your goals. With monitors readily available and inexpensive, there is no reason anyone should not use one.

Know Your Heart

Once you know your heart rate, you can train in specific zones tailored to your goals for that training period. Each zone corresponds to a heart rate range relative to your maximum heart rate. Aerobic conditioning takes place when training keeps your heart rate between 70 percent and 80 percent of your max heart rate. Anaerobic conditioning takes place when training keeps your heart rate between 80 percent and 90 percent of your max heart rate. Training above 90 percent of your maximum heart rate can only be maintained for short periods of time.

There are many heart rate monitors on the market. Some simply tell you your current heart rate, while others allow you to connect to your computer so you can record and download your heart rate and give you a summary for each training period. Some monitors will even allow you to set the type of workout you are going to do and then warn you when you are above or below your target heart rate. Prices range from $29 to over $500.

Aerobic Training

Aerobic training conditions the cardiopulmonary system—your heart and lungs. Specific attention must be paid to aerobic training since it provides support for all effort lasting more than two minutes. The blood pumped by your heart transports oxygen and nutrients into your muscle cells while transporting waste away from them. Your muscles cannot perform beyond the limits of your cardiopulmonary system's performance capacity.

Your aerobic capacity will dictate not only the time duration but also the intensity at which you are capable of exercising (which often translates over into your performance in a fight). Poor aerobic fitness means slower and longer recovery periods between flurries of strikes, between rounds, and between workouts.

116

Immediate Physiological Effects

After the first two minutes of training, the period when you start to burn stored glycogen for energy, aerobic training is the most important factor affecting your performance. In Krav Maga classes you acquire your aerobic training in fitness classes where you perform combinations of punches and kicks for twenty to sixty minutes.

Shadowboxing is clearly sport specific, giving you an opportunity to hone your combative techniques. In the environment of a fitness class, some techniques may have to be shortchanged to keep up with the speed of the class. This doesn't mean you should avoid them, just be aware. Shadowboxing at your own pace doesn't have this drawback.

Anaerobic Training

Anaerobic training helps develop your ability to perform very intensely for short period of time. The difference between aerobic and anaerobic has to do with the source of energy used. Each must be distinctly trained to develop their unique qualities.

Exercise lasting less than thirty seconds relies on the phosphagen system. Between thirty seconds and two minutes of exercise, energy is supplied by utilizing phosphagen and lactic acid. The goal of interval training is to increase our anaerobic capacity by improving the use of these energy systems and increasing our tolerance to lactic acid in the muscles.

You use interval training to develop your anaerobic capacity. Interval training requires short periods of effort (punching and kicking, swimming, sprinting) at near maximum capacity. An anaerobic interval is simply a period of training between 30 and 120 seconds. Intervals can be performed by themselves (thirty-second sprints with a period of rest in between), or they can be mixed into a more comprehensive workout (a number of thirty-second sprints performed within a five-mile run).

Interval Training for Best Results

Our bodies must be efficient at providing energy for each zone. Interval training develops aerobic capacity as well as anaerobic conditioning without the deleterious effects on muscle that extensive aerobic training can have. Training exclusively and extensively in the aerobic zone leads to muscle loss and corresponding losses in speed and power.

Next time you watch a track and field event, notice the physical differences between the short-distance runners and the long-distance runners.

How do you supply your muscles with the energy to fight, train, or perform everyday or sport-specific activities? Your body generates energy from three sources—phosphagen, glycogen, and oxygen—based on the effort and duration of the task. You consume glycogen and phosphagen, and your body absorbs oxygen through the lungs and skin from your surrounding environment.

Phosphagen is used in the very initial stages of exercise, the first ten seconds, and powers highly intense effort. To train this energy system:

1. Train intensely for 10–30 seconds.
2. Rest and recover for three times as long as you worked.
3. Repeat 5–10 times.

EXAMPLE: Do a twenty-second sprint, rest for sixty seconds, and repeat five times. Then immediately do twenty seconds of pushups (as many as you can in that period), rest for sixty seconds, repeat five times, and then repeat the sprints for a total of three intervals.

Glycogen is used for moderately intense exercise that lasts for two to three minutes. To train your glycogen pathways you should:

1. Work up to 6–8 intervals.
2. Rest for twice as long as you worked.

EXAMPLE: Do one minute of hard shadowboxing or punching and kicking on a heavy bag, then rest for two minutes. Repeat six to eight times.

Oxygen is used for relatively easy exercise that lasts longer than several minutes. To train your oxygen energy source:

1. Train at an easy to moderate intensity of 10–60 minute sets for an equivalent period (three minutes) of time.
2. Repeat 5 times.

Phosphagen and glycogen are gained and utilized through anaerobic exercise, while oxygen is gained and utilized through aerobic exercise. You must train in the use of all of these energy sources in order to be truly fit. In the context of a fight, you might make it through the first round with good anaerobic conditioning, but unless you score a first round knockout, you will need equally good aerobic conditioning to make it through the rest of the fight.

Krav Maga training uses continuous full-power combinations of combatives and techniques to build anaerobic capacity. These can be isolated drills or used within longer sessions of shadowboxing.

Cross Training

Cross training means using a variety of training methods within a workout. In general, cross training helps keep your workouts interesting and balanced. Once you determine the goals of your workout (in the larger context of your overall plan), you can mix aerobic and anaerobic training, strength, endurance, core, and sport-specific movements into a single workout, circuits, and intervals. By combining different training methods you can achieve the benefits of certain methods or movements while negating their shortcomings.

Mixing It Up

Different training methods combine to give the best overall results. Sport-specific drills are necessary, but in the case of fighting, it would probably be too hard on the body to train three hours a day, six days a week, via full contact sparring.

So along with some sparring, also do weight training, running, and plyometrics. This allows you to wear yourself out (without overtraining) yet continue to build strength, endurance, power, and coordination.

If at some point it becomes a burden to keep lifting weights, you can do slow training on technique. When you can no longer do another pushup, switch to squats. This enables you to keep building your body beyond what you could accomplish with only one training method.

FACT

A variety of training reduces the risk of overtraining, which requires time off to recover, and reduces the risk of joint injuries from continuously repeating the same motion.

The Importance of Cross Training

Cross training keeps your body from getting used to a particular training method, helping to break or avoid training plateaus (periods of slow or no improvement). It may also allow you to have more intense workouts by working different groups of muscles from one workout to the next.

A fighter will use all of the above training methods, combined with proper nutrition and adequate sleep, to get into fighting shape. Workouts will build up to the point where training takes place twice a day for two to four hours at a time. They will include sport-specific training drills to develop strong and fast combatives and defensive techniques, actual sparring, and strength training. Cross training is the only way to maintain the intensity and endurance to complete the workouts.

Bike, Run, Swim

A triathlete is, by definition, someone who does a lot of cross training. Cross training can be done within a single workout or by rotating through different types of workouts. The nice thing about this combination is the variety of muscles, movements, and energy sources involved. It's also really nice to get a little fresh air and sunshine while you exercise, but depending on where you live these may not be year-round activities.

Cycling

Cycling is a fine way to push your cardio without additional impact to your bones and joints. Maintain a steady ninety revolutions per minute, adjusting the resistance to maintain the desired heart rate. Use interval training (short-distance sprints) to add anaerobic development to the work out. With cycling you have the option of working within your aerobic or anaerobic ranges, in a spinning class at the local gym, or mountain biking. Mountain biking requires move overall coordination and strength.

Running

Running is part of every fighter's training routine. Run at a pace that allows you to carry on a conversation. Every few minutes, break into a twenty- to forty-second sprint, and then slow to a jog while you recover, then begin running again.

ALERT

With regard to cycling and running, you should be conscientious of repetitive stress injuries and the wear and tear on some joints.

Remember to approach your training program holistically, that is, as a whole with the end in mind. If you are training for a mixed martial arts (MMA) fight, you'll need a combination of aerobic and anaerobic conditioning, enough to maintain an intense level for as little as two five-minute rounds or as much as three ten-minute rounds. You will need to be explosive for unpredictable intervals during this time. So it makes no sense to train only long-distance runs. This will detract from other areas, making it difficult, if not impossible, to also maintain strength and explosiveness. The goal is to maximize aerobic and anaerobic improvement, so mix it up.

Swimming

Swimming, another low-impact exercise, has some special benefits. The movements you make while swimming require lengthening the muscles and the body overall as opposed to the compression that most other training applies. This helps improve flexibility and range of motion. It also places additional demands on the cardio system because you now need to control your breathing relative to external influences (so you don't choke on the water).

Different strokes can place more emphasis on certain muscles, but swimming works the entire body, especially the core muscles needed to move the arms and legs in unison.

Plyometrics

Plyometrics fall into the resistance category, using your own body weight as the resistance. Plyometrics are effective for body control because they build explosive power, strength, balance, and coordination. In terms of everyday fitness, plyometric conditioning is the most useful and appropriate type of training. When added into a workout that includes cardio conditioning, you have a complete regimen.

Plyometrics don't require any equipment and can be done in a relatively small space, so they are useful for those who travel, work out in at the office, or for anyone who gets the sudden urge to work on conditioning.

Plyometric exercises include pushups (perform the pushup so explosively that your body and hands leave the ground), Jumping Squats, and Jumping Lunges. For more on plymometrics, see Chapter 7.

Circuit Training

A circuit is simply a series of exercises designed to simultaneously develop strength or sport-specific skills and cardiovascular conditioning. Circuit training develops both aerobic and anaerobic capacity by including short bursts of effort in the context of a longer overall series of exercises.

Circuit Example 1

The following example combines aerobic and anaerobic conditioning, strength training, interval training, cross training, plyometrics, and sport-specific conditioning.

1. 400 meter run (quarter mile)
2. 30 seconds of slow, controlled pushups
3. 30 seconds of Jumping Lunges
4. 30 seconds of continuous full-power punches to a heavy bag

You should have a minimal resting period between sets while on any one circuit, with a longer two-minute rest between circuits. ■

Circuit Example 2

1. 30 seconds of Basic Squats with the medicine ball (Chapter 6, page 66).
2. 30 seconds of alternating Lunges with ball overhead (Chapter 5, page 51).
3. 30 seconds of Russian Twists (Chapter 16, page 192).
4. 30 seconds of face-up Cross Extensions (Chapter 16, page 191).
5. Light shadowboxing for 1 minute.
6. Repeat.

You may repeat a circuit a few times or perform different circuits. ■

11 INJURY AND INJURY PREVENTION

As with any sport or activity, when the intensity of training goes up, unfortunately so does the chance of injury. This is why it's important to become aware of how and why injuries occur within a Krav Maga training program in order to avoid them. Some injuries are specific to Krav Maga, and other injuries can happen within any training program. This chapter will discuss injuries, explain how you can do your best to prevent injuries from occurring, and the best ways to treat them if and when they do occur.

Good Pain Versus Bad Pain

It's important to know what kind of pain you are dealing with when exercising. Many sedentary people associate exercise with pain. It's important to keep in mind that muscle fatigue is not the same as pain, which is a result of compression of a joint, excessive tension in a tendon, or a torn ligament. There is a certain degree of discomfort within an exercise, but that discomfort should not feel like sharp pain near or within a joint region. If you do feel sharp pain with a movement or exercise, you should stop immediately and evaluate where the pain is coming from and what is causing it. Be sure to contact a doctor or health professional if the pain is persistent or if it worsens.

Injuries fall into two categories. *Acute* injuries are caused by an immediate trauma, such as stepping off a curb and rolling your ankle. *Chronic* injuries are generally developed over time and result from overuse with repetitive actions such as throwing, running, or jumping. Although an acute injury can happen at any time, whether you are playing sports or not, if you are training in a safe environment and progress your exercises appropriately you should not experience a traumatic injury during training.

Common Types of Injuries

It is very rare to come across an adult who is not dealing with some sort of repetitive stress syndrome. It's a part of life. You need to recognize the movements you do repetitively due to the lifestyle you live and treat those areas of the body with respect.

INFLAMMATION: For most people this word has a negative connotation. It is important to remember that inflammation is an integral part of the healing process. When tissues are damaged or irritated, inflammation must occur for the healing process to begin. Tissues become damaged, then swelling and inflammation occurs in the damaged area to promote healing. This is an appropriate response and a good thing for the body to do. However, it is supposed to be a short process that ends when healing has been accomplished. If the source of the problem (irritation and overuse) does not recede, then the inflammatory process may become a painful and chronic condition.

TENDONITIS: The most commonly reported overuse injury is tendonitis. The suffix *-itis* means "inflammation." So, tendonitis means inflammation of the tendon. As bodies move, tendons slide and rub over the structures that surround them.

124

When a movement is repeated, the rubbing and sliding irritates the tendon causing pain and swelling. Warmth is often associated with that swelling. The best way to treat tendonitis is to rest. It's recommended to rest the irritated area for two weeks. However, athletes and regular exercisers find it hard to stop training for two weeks. You should try to find an alternative exercise for that period of time. This is when cross training can be beneficial. If you like to run, you may try swimming or cycling for a couple of weeks. Try to choose an activity that does not stress the irritated joint in the same way.

BURSITIS: Within the joints of the human body are fluid-filled sacs called bursae. The function of these bursae are to cushion, reduce friction, and lubricate joints to allow for smooth movements. There are about 160 bursae throughout the body, and they are found in regions such as the hips, knees, shoulders, and elbows. If excessive movement or trauma occurs to a joint or around a bursa sac, it can become irritated or inflamed. When the bursa becomes irritated, it produces synovial fluid to protect the area. If the irritation persists, the accumulation of fluid in the joint capsule begins to create pressure that can restrict movement and become very painful.

The most commonly irritated bursae are found in the shoulder and the knee. The best thing to do for bursitis is to rest the affected joint and ice the irritated area. It may help to take an over-the-counter pain killer or anti-inflammatory.

OSTEOARTHRITIS: Any mechanical system that is used frequently will inevitably show signs of wear and tear. The same holds true for the joints within the body. The body is a mechanical system and is constantly being worn down, even with normal activity. Wear and tear of a joint usually results in a degeneration of the cartilage found within the joint. When this cartilage is worn away the underlying bone can be exposed, which causes a great deal of pain. The best way to nurse a condition such as this is to rest the affected area to alleviate the pain and keep the joints strong so they continue to have a good support system. Some experts recommend a low-impact stretching program that will help create space between the joints, which may decrease the forces of compression.

Acute Injuries

Acute injuries are injuries that occur immediately, and they can be rated from mild to severe. For example, you can have from mild sprain to a ligament in the knee in which case you may feel some pain, but with ice and rest it will return to normal. On the other hand, you may see a much more severe injury to a ligament in the knee in which surgery is sometimes necessary.

When implementing the Krav Maga fitness program appropriately, it is not likely that you will experience a severe injury such as this. Though injury is always a possibility, the longer you train, the less likely you are to have one. If anything, a program such as Krav Maga is going to aid you in preventing these types of injuries.

Muscles

Muscle tissue is made up of fibers that are capable of lengthening and shortening. They have a certain amount of elasticity to them, and if they are forced past the point of elasticity it is possible to separate or tear the fibers. This damage is referred to as a strain. Each muscle is attached to the bones by a tendon. Tendon tissue is not nearly as elastic as muscle tissue, so when the muscle is lengthened past the point of no return, the region where the injury is most likely to occur is where the muscle and tendon meet. Muscle strains are classified into a simple system:

- *Grade 1 strain*: Some of the fibers have been stretched past their limit or mildly torn. Although there is tenderness and pain with movement, it is possible to move the area without limitations. Usually ice and rest will help a grade 1 strain recover.
- *Grade 2 strain*: Many of the muscle fibers have been torn and it is painful when the muscle actively contracts. Many times a depression can be felt where the injury occurred. There may be some swelling or discoloration due to the capillaries being damaged. This injury is more severe and will take much more time to heal than a grade 1 strain. In this case it is beneficial to wrap the injured area with an ace bandage. Ice, elevation, and compression are needed. It may help to see a doctor for an examination and x-ray to be sure nothing else is damaged.
- *Grade 3 strain*: This involves a complete tear of the muscle or tendon tissue. With a complete tear there is a loss of movement. Initially this is very painful, but the pain may diminish due to the nerve fiber being separated. A great deal of discoloration will occur. This injury should been seen by a doctor immediately.

Muscle Soreness

Although you are not likely to experience any severe injuries in the Krav Maga program, one of the most common minor acute injuries you should be aware of is muscle soreness. A certain level of soreness is inevitable when beginning a training program, or when doing an exercise to which you are not accustomed. There are two types of muscle soreness. The first is the soreness you feel immediately after an exercise, which usually is accompanied by fatigue. The second is known as *delayed onset of muscle soreness*, or DOMS, which is most intense after twenty-four to forty-eight hours and gradually subsides over a few days. This soreness is thought to be caused by microscopic tears or damage to the muscles and tendons from being overworked, and it can lead to swelling and stiffness.

Muscle soreness can't be prevented, but it can be lessened by implementing a proper warm-up and increasing the intensity of your training sessions slowly over time. You can treat muscle soreness with light activity. Twenty to thirty minutes of light to moderate cardiorespiratory exercise can help the body feel loosened up, and the increase of blood flow can decrease the amount of pain felt. Some experts recommend stretching as a modality, and even ice. If the pain inhibits you from performing daily activity, you may take an over-the-counter painkiller such as ibuprofen or acetaminophen.

Muscle Cramps

Muscle cramps are very common among athletes, avid exercisers, and individuals in the beginning stages of an exercise program. Cramps are involuntary muscle contractions that can occur in any muscle but are most common in the feet, calves, hamstrings, and abdominal musculature. Very little is known about cramps and why they occur, but research indicates cramps occur due to loss of electrolytes such as sodium, calcium, potassium, and magnesium, which are all essential in muscle contraction. When a cramp comes on, the best thing to do is relax the muscle as much as possible. Take some deep breaths, calm yourself down, and drink plenty of fluids to rehydrate your body. Some experts recommend massage and stretching the muscle that has cramped.

Contusions

A contusion is a fancy name for a bruise. Bruising is usually caused by a blow from an outside object. Krav Maga is a contact activity, so it is likely that some bruising will occur. This is common in the beginning stages so don't be alarmed. Try to keep your punches and kicks light until you feel your technique is developed. Once you use the correct alignment, the bruising will diminish and you can make stronger contact without turning black and blue the next day.

Ligaments

Ligaments attach bone to bone and provide support to joints. Ligament tissue is relatively inelastic, unlike muscle tissue that lengthens easily. If a joint is moved or forced beyond its limits, injury to a ligament is likely to occur. The greatest problem with trauma to a ligament is that ligament tissue has very limited blood supply so it takes a long time to heal. And once a ligament as been stretched, scar tissue begins to form which limits the ligament's ability to return to its original tension. This makes it hard to restore stability to the joint. The best thing to do is to strengthen the tendons and muscles surrounding the joint to provide added stability where it has been lost. As with muscle strains, ligament strains are also classified into a system that determines the severity of the injury.

Ligament Sprain Grading Scale

- *Grade 1 sprain*: Some stretching and separation of the ligaments fibers has occurred. There may be a slight amount of instability to the joint. There may be mild pain and swelling. Joint stiffness should be expected. Rest, ice, compression, and elevation are the best ways to treat a grade 1 sprain.

- *Grade 2 sprain*: Some tearing and separation occurs within the ligament and moderate instability of the joint is noticeable. Pain is moderate to severe with a grade 2 sprain. Swelling and joint stiffness is evident. Again, rest, ice, elevate, and compress the injury. It may be a good choice to have a doctor examine the injury to be sure no other damage has occurred.

- *Grade 3 Sprain*: This is a total tearing of the ligament and major instability of the joint is apparent. Initially, pain is severe and will subside due to nerves being disrupted. A great deal of swelling will be present, and the joint tends to become very stiff. A grade 3 sprain will often require surgical repair. Usually with an injury as severe as this, other injuries will occur, such as a bone fracture or muscle damage. Get to your doctor immediately for a thorough examination of the injury.

Applying ice immediately after any sprain will greatly increase your chances for recovery.

ALERT

Do not apply ice directly to the skin or you put yourself at risk for frostbite. Use a towel between the ice and the injury, or use an ice bag. Apply ice for twenty minutes at a time, with at least twenty minutes between applications.

128

The Common Aches and Pains of Krav Maga

The most common joints that receive repetitive stress from an ongoing Krav Maga training program are the shoulders, elbows, knees, wrists, and lower back. It is important to keep these joints strong in order to avoid aches and pains that may go along with this type of training. When performing punches repetitively, the shoulder and elbow have to do a lot of work to extend punches out and back. When making contact to a bag or pad when punching, you then add an additional force into the equation. When making contact, the wrist absorbs a large amount of force from compression, which is distributed up through the bones of your arm. This force can seriously jar your shoulder.

When the punch is delivered with proper mechanics, it is less likely to cause an injury. Just as important, the bones and connective tissues have to adapt to the impact that goes along with punching. You should always start slowly, even if you have perfect mechanics, and progress speed and strength appropriately.

Some Krav Maga students report pain in their lower backs from repetitive round kicks to a bag or pad. This might be due to the fact that their muscles are not yet strong enough to support the force they are generating to deliver strong round kicks. This is why it's important that you keep joints and connective tissues strong, not only for a healthy back but to sustain the force of the kicks you will be delivering. You need to keep your spine strong and mobile in order to move well.

The best way to avoid aches and pains in the commonly stressed joints from Krav Maga training is to keep joints strong and flexible. This way you have the ability to move through the proper ROM without forcing mechanics, and you have enough strength to support the force being generated.

Preventing Injuries

So what are the best exercises to keep the joints strong to prevent injuries before they occur? The following functional training exercises are some of the best exercises to keep joints flexible and strong at the same time.

Injury Preventions Steps

- *Exercising the feet and ankles*: The feet are the foundation of your entire body, so it's important to have healthy, strong feet. Usually the arches will collapse because of weakness in the foot. With you shoes off, work on spreading your toes away from each other as much as possible. You can do this while watching TV. The toe spread can also be done while standing upright. It's a great exercise to strengthen you feet. To strengthen your ankles, practice rolling your ankles around slowly with full range of motion. Pay attention to all the muscles in the lower leg that have to contract and lengthen in order to make the ankle move with such control.

- *Healthy knees and hips*: A great deal of the muscles that are part of the hip are also part of the knee. A Basic Squat (Chapter 6, page 66) can strengthen the hips and the knees. Once you are comfortable with a Basic Squat, work on full squats. This increases the range of motion in the hips and knees as well as increases strength through that range of motion. Lunges of all types are also a great way to increase strength through range of motion. Functional training exercises can also be done as part of an injury prevention plan for your hips and knees.

- *Protect the shoulders*: The shoulder joint is a very fragile joint. It has the ability to perform very large movements in an infinite amount of directions. It is often thought as a ball and socket joint, but this is a misconception. What holds the shoulder joint in place is the rotator cuff complex. This small group of muscles has to be strengthened in all Krav Maga students in order to maintain a healthy shoulder. Anything that involves rotation with some kind of resistance against it will help to strengthen this muscle group.

- *Healthy back and spine*: There are many exercises that promote a healthy back and spine. All of the exercises that are included in the core training chapter can strengthen the back and spine and keep it mobile. The spine rotates, flexes forward, extends back, and bends laterally. All of these movements need to be done to stay mobile and strong, so it is essential that core training be done to promote this. Exercises such as the Cobra (Chapter 5, page 53), Downward Facing Dog (Chapter 5, page 50), Plank (Chapter 16, page 188), Cross Extensions (Chapter 16, page 191), and Leg Lifts (Chapter 8, page 101) are beneficial movements that need to be continuously practiced.

Overtraining and Exercise Burnout

There is a difference between overtraining and exercise burnout, and sometimes it can be a bit confusing. Overtraining is when athletes or individuals who exercise frequently expose themselves to excessive amounts of training that are near or at max levels of intensity. Some of the symptoms of overtraining include physical and mental exhaustion, poor heart rate recovery, depression, sleep disturbances, and irritability.

Overtraining can also affect athletic performance. Usually when one is overtraining, muscles become fatigued and cannot fire as quickly and efficiently. Strength and endurance decreases, and you may experience negative mood changes, which can then lead to burnout.

Physical and Emotional Burnout

Exercise burnout involves an emotional and sometimes physical withdrawal from a previously enjoyable activity due to excessive stress or dissatisfaction over a period of time. Some of the signs or symptoms of burnout are loss of interest and energy, feelings of low accomplishment, low self-esteem, and feeling like a failure. Ignoring these symptoms usually results in an individual quitting training. It is important to notice the signs and treat them appropriately.

Burnout and overtraining are prevented and treated the same way. It is essential for one's health and well-being to take time off from jobs and any other stressors in life. This is why you have weekends, holidays, and vacation time. The same holds true for exercise. It is fine to take time to train lightly or not at all so the mental and physical systems of the body can recover appropriately. Without proper recovery of the mind and body, the risk of injury increases substantially.

Dealing with Burnout

So what do you do? Get a massage or treat yourself to a day at the spa. Another great way to prevent burnout is to take a gentle yoga class that emphasizes deep breathing. Many athletes learn how to meditate or practice visualization techniques in order to relax. This can help with everyday stress as well. Communication is another way to deal will stress. Talk to friends, family, or even a therapist. Having a social support system to express your feelings can help alleviate frustrations, anxiety, and disappointment. Keep a positive outlook even if things are getting tough. It is a common in life to have ups and downs. Remember, even when the going gets tough and the moment feels like it's never-ending, look back and be satisfied and proud of your accomplishments. Remember these tips for preventing injuries and burnout:

- Increase time and intensity gradually
- Properly hydrate your body
- Warm up properly
- Listen to your body
- Cross train
- Rest when needed
- Eat appropriately
- Treat yourself to a massage
- Meditate

131

12 INTRODUCTION TO FUNCTIONAL TRAINING

Functional training involves working combinations of muscles and joints as opposed to simply working on isolated muscles. It emphasizes the inclusion of trunk and core muscles in order to train the body to move more efficiently by not wasting any exerted energy. A well-designed functional training program will use a variety of movements that coordinate the use of both the upper and lower extremities, while focusing on sharpening your ability to initiate movement from the midsection of the body (your core).

Functional Training

Functional training is a whole-body training method that involves working combinations of muscles and joints, as opposed to simply working on isolated muscles, while emphasizing the inclusion of trunk and core muscles in order to train the body to move more efficiently.

Why is functional training important? When performing exercises such as punches and kicks, the body is continuously moving a number of parts simultaneously. The arms, legs, and torso of the body are forced to move in a coordinated sequence, which can become rather exhausting very quickly.

For instance, in order to strengthen the power of your punches, you wouldn't spend all of your time building up your deltoid (shoulder) muscles. For increased punching power, you also need to strengthen the muscles in your chest, back, core, and legs.

Moving Your Body Effectively

In order for your body to perform an effective punch, be it a hook or a straight jab, all of the necessary muscles must work together. Rather than training all of these muscles individually (which would take a very long time), it would make far more sense to perform multilimb exercise movements. Functional training exercises strengthen your entire body as a whole.

One example of a strength-training exercise in which both the legs and arms are used together is holding a weighted or medicine ball (see Chapter 7, page 87) while performing a combined exercise of a Basic Squat (Chapter 6, page 66) with an overhead lift of the ball. This exercise directly strengthens a myriad of muscle groups while developing a coordinated movement pattern that will aid the body in becoming more mechanically efficient.

Accustomed to Symmetry

Your body can become too accustomed to symmetrical patterns of motion, primarily because a majority of your regular functions (such as walking) require such movements. With each step, your body performs opposite but symmetrically similar movements— one foot goes back while the other goes forward, one arms swing back while the other comes up.

Exercises that work the limbs together will help develop coordination, which will translate into making complex movements (like the Hook Punch in Chapter 13, page 153 or Side Kick in Chapter 14, page 166) feel more natural and fluid. This will ease the transition of both your mind and body as you encounter more mechanically complex techniques later on in your training.

Fitness for the Everyday Battles

Not only does functional training enhance sports performance, but it also makes everyday activities more efficient. Functional training will increase your ability to perform normal everyday activities such as carrying groceries up a flight of stairs, placing a weighted object on a high shelf, or lifting heavy objects up off the floor. Functional training exercises can make these tasks feel much easier and less stressful on your muscles and joints. It also decreases your risk of injury from performing these tasks.

Functional training enhances activities in different sports. An athlete from any sport will be able to increase his or her level of performance by implementing a functional training routine. However, a golfer may not necessarily increase the distance of his or her drive by doing the intensive footwork and speed training that you would likely see a football player doing. In Krav Maga, functional training exercises are used to increase the power and improve the performance of punches, kicks, body weight shifts, and body movement in a coordinated and controlled manner.

Sport-Specific Training

Sport-specific training exercises are movements that mimic or resemble as closely as possible the athletic needs of the individual trainee based upon the physical demands that are placed upon her by her selected sport.

In Krav Maga, conditioning movements that are similar (and therefore beneficial) to certain techniques are exercises such as:

- *Pushups*—Simulates the action of punching (Chapter 16, page 188)
- *Leg swings*—Swinging one leg forward and up in front of you simulates what the leg would be doing when delivering a kick.
- *Bob and weave drills*—By learning to bend at the knees and hips to lower the head so as to avoid a punch, these drills teach you how to properly move your head and shift your bodyweight in order to put together effective combinations of punches and kicks. When working to the focus mitts it's important to move like you would be moving in a fight. The bobbing action is moving the head straight down and up by bending at the knees and waist slightly as if to duck underneath a punch. The weaving action is moving the either right or left to dodge a punch. When you put the two together you are perfoming a bob and weave. This is a great exercise to train proper head and body movement when training combatives.

The Effects of Timing on Training

Not only does sport-specific training relate to the mechanics of the activity, but it relates to the intensity and duration required for the activity. For example, a sprinter is obviously going to need a somewhat different training regime than a marathon runner. It simply would not make sense for an athlete who needs to be able to perform at very high-intensity levels for somewhat short bursts to have a training regime that consisted of jogging for long periods of time. The opposite would be true for endurance or marathon runners, as their needs are based upon a prolonged pace instead of on short, intense bursts of speed.

ESSENTIAL

Creativity is a big part of sport-specific training. Know your activity and train for it. For example, an Olympic fencer needs to be light and fast, as well as quick and accurate at lunging. Strong wrists along with powerful but flexible leg muscles are essential for such an athlete. Therefore, it would not make a lot of sense for an Olympic fencer to cross train in power lifting.

For Krav Maga, sport-specific takes on a new meaning. Krav Maga is about self-defense and dealing with the unexpected at a moment's notice. This includes learning to hit your competition mode faster in response to situational changes, with little to no warning, when you encounter them in an uncontrolled environment.

Krav Maga and Functional Training

Most Krav Maga training centers and gyms offer fitness classes in addition to their self-defense and fighting classes. These are both functional as well as sport-specific training programs. These classes are specifically designed to improve the practitioner's overall health as well as mental and physical conditioning while improving his Krav Maga skills. For a list of locations and contact information of KMAA facilities, please refer to Appendix A.

Athletes need to train in ways that simulate the environments in which they play their sports. That being said, Krav Maga is based on defending yourself on the street, or wherever such a need may arise. An unfamiliar or unexpected environment can ambush you just as effectively as an unseen opponent. For example:

- *Parking lots*: You have to be aware not to stumble over parking blocks, get yourself backed into a light post, or end up trapped between two cars.
- *Stairwells*: There is a limited amount of space in which to move, only two directions of advance or retreat, and you have to maneuver on an uneven platform.
- *Bars or nightclubs*: These places are very crowded, making it easy for opponents to disappear from your sight and reappear to attack you from another angle as they lose themselves in a sea of people.

Finding Environments for Functional Training

Whatever the situation may be, an unfamiliar environment can affect your focus and decrease the efficiency of your defense. What the Krav Maga practitioner needs to be aware of while training is that although she may be in a safe and controlled environment that has tremendous benefits, it is also important to train under a variety of simulated conditions. Doing so will teach your body to be aware of and adjust for different surroundings.

FACT

Training in environments that you are likely to encounter danger is important in Krav Maga. If you only train in environments where you feel comfortable, then you may find yourself at a disadvantage when confronted with violence in an unfamiliar environment.

The following are different environments and situations to try:

- *Dark room*: Learning to move about in a dark room will help you learn to compensate with your other senses after a sudden loss of light or eyesight. For example, people tend to attack at chest level when they can't see an opponent, so you may find it beneficial to crouch.
- *Parking lots or public parks*: Sprinting in bursts through a parking lot, moving suddenly from concrete to grass, or cutting across a parking lot of loose gravel will help your speed and balance.

- *Loud music*: Training with extremely loud music will teach you to think and compensate with your other senses for a sudden loss of hearing due to noise from a loud car horn, a noisy bar, or concert speakers.
- *Crowded areas*: Have you ever found yourself out of breath after crossing a crowded room? The bodies that surround you in a crowd offer resistance against the direction you choose to move. Learning to run or walk through a crowd offers more than just a workout, it teaches you to maneuver and aids you in overcoming the claustrophobia or disorientation these situations can cause in an emergency.
- *With groceries and/or car keys in your hands*: Being confronted by an attacker while holding an armful of groceries is probably one of the most vulnerable feelings that any one could experience, which means you should be prepared for it.
- *Stairwells*: Running up and down on both outdoor and enclosed stairwells is great for increasing leg muscle and cardiovascular endurance. It will also familiarize you with the limited side-to-side (or other directional) mobility of such an environment.

Functional Drills

Among other things, Krav Maga students need to practice drills in order to learn the basic footwork necessary to be both a good martial artist and an effective fighter. In Chapter 18 you will learn practice drills that condition you to employ speed, agility, coordination, balance, and power in an attack. With these drills, you can practice various combinations of punches and kicks, at a number of different speeds and angles, in order to train your body to perform these techniques correctly and effectively without having to consciously think about every single move as you transition from one technique to the next.

As a Krav Maga practitioner, you should strive to reach the point where the body's movements happen with as little thought as possible, nearly effortless, so that you can focus on becoming stronger in your body and sharper and more aware in your mind, all the while keeping yourself safe from harm and ill health.

Training for the Competitive Fighter

Punching, kicking, and moving in different combinations while not leaving yourself open to an opponent's attack should be a goal in your training. Such abilities are what competitive fighters train for, and it's what you should be practicing in your Krav Maga training. The key is to emphasize different aspects of your primary techniques in order to intelligently balance development of your skills.

For example, varying the speed at which you train improves different aspects of your overall performance. Slow work will build on your technique and balance, while powerful strokes to a heavy bag will build your strength and punching power. Concentrating on the speed of your recoil (an action which follows just about every striking technique) will aid you in building rapid combinations of fast strikes, which are covered in Chapter 18.

ESSENTIAL

Professional fighters are among the most highly conditioned athletes in the world. For today's mixed martial arts fighters, a fight could last as long as thirty minutes, and in some arenas the fight lasts until someone wins. This means that these fighters have to maintain a constant level of physical fitness (or level of endurance) in order to stay competitive with their opponents.

The Fitness of Fighters

Professional or competitive fighters should be in a relatively high level of fitness at all times and will rarely have long offseasons as professional athletes such as baseball or football players. Professional fighters build to a peak level over a six- to ten-week period that is reached only a few nights to a week prior to the actual fight.

138

It is quite common for a professional fighter to train in the gym for three to four hours at a time, two times a day, over several weeks. Of course, a proper diet and a steady sleeping cycle are essential elements in maintaining this intense pace of training for such an extended period of time. For more information on diet and nutrition, please refer to Chapter 3. Low blood sugar levels, electrolyte imbalances, or even the slightest infection of the body can spell disaster for a competitive fighter.

Training for Every Round

When an athlete is training for a fight, the most crucial piece of information that her trainer needs to know is how long the match is going to last—how many rounds total and the length of the rounds. A boxing match can be anywhere from three to ten rounds, ranging from two to three minutes each. But mixed martial arts (MMA) or no-holds-barred (NHB) matches are often two to five rounds with anywhere from five- to fifteen-minute rounds.

Whatever the length of the rounds, the possibility that the fighter will go the whole duration of the fight (which for MMA fighters can mean a total fight time of over an hour) needs to be accounted for in the training regime. In fact, it would be ideal if that time is slightly exceeded during training to ensure that the fighter can meet the highest potential for physical demands the fight could have.

This way the fighter learns how to pace herself. The fighter will build both the strength and endurance needed in order to effectively fight for as many rounds as is necessary. As any fighter or trainer will tell you, whenever you have a fight between two fighters who are nearly equal in skill level and experience, the the winner is often the fighter that trained harder. It all comes down to conditioning. On the street, where there are no rounds, conditioning may be the only advantage you have when facing a larger attacker.

For the Beginner Krav Maga Student

A new Krav Maga student should begin training for an average of sixty minutes, two to three times per week. This time frame should include all of the basic components of the training session:

- Warm-up
- Strength training
- Stretching
- Krav Maga combative drills
- Cool down

ALERT

Don't try to do it all when you are at the beginning stages of your training. Overdoing things in the beginning will lead to soreness, fatigue, and possibly injury. There is nothing wrong with pushing yourself, but be aware of your limits when you first begin training.

New Krav Maga students have to remember to keep their exercises simple in order to learn the correct movement patterns of their joints and muscles. At the outset of your experience with any martial arts or fight training, learning how to punch, kick, block, or even how to just stand up properly can make you feel quite awkward. (For some it can be the most awkward feelings they have ever experienced.) This can cause frustration for beginners, which can lead to a lack of motivation to continue with their training. There is a secret to overcome this first and often most difficult hurdle in your Krav Maga training: Don't give up!

QUESTION

How do I overcome the temptation to give up when things get rough in the beginning of my Krav Maga training?
Try to always keep in mind your reasons for wanting to train. It also helps to set goals, because when things get tough you can think, "If I quit now, I'll never reach my goals." Motivation and intensity are big parts of Krav Maga training, and your mind is going to be taxed just as much as your body in order to assure that, when the time comes for you to stand and fight, you do not panic.

Learning to Act Natural

Krav Maga does not require any particularly difficult or unnatural movements. On the contrary, its whole premise is using natural and instinctive movements. With just a few days of practice on any given technique, the movements will become less awkward for you. Your body will begin to adapt to movements that at first had felt very foreign. You will begin to feel yourself becoming considerably more comfortable, executing your techniques better and better with each Krav Maga class and training session that you complete.

Newer students often have a tendency to become fatigued far sooner than more advanced students. This is, for the most part, simply a matter of conditioning as new students adjust to the mental stress and energy required to learn and practice Krav Maga. Less-experienced students have not yet learned how to execute these movements as efficiently as those who have more training time and experience under their belts. In just a short time, you will be able to relax your mind and body as the movements become patterns in your nervous system, requiring less conscious thought to perform.

Remember to Breathe

Breathing may seem like an obvious necessity, but it takes some practice to do properly while training or performing under stress. Expelling air as you expend energy helps relax the body and, more importantly, forces you to breathe in. Nothing will fatigue you more quickly than the lack of oxygen. So if at any time you begin feeling as though you are short of breath while working with intensity, focus on making your inhales deeper and controlling your exhales. Learning to do this will help you to stay calm, recover more quickly, and continue moving. Proper breathing patterns are discussed in Chapter 5.

> ### ALERT
>
> Avoid tensing up your body! Rigidity in the body means slower reaction time and may cause you to telegraph your movements, giving your opponent cues to dodge and/or block your attacks. A crucial element to becoming an effective fighter is learning to maintain a relaxed yet aware posture. The more rigid your body is, the more unnecessary energy it is going to exert and the higher your risk of injury will be.

For all these reasons, beginners often have a hard time maintaining a high level of intensity during their first few weeks of Krav Maga classes. Rest assured that your body will adjust quickly to the new demands you place upon it, as long as you are willing and able to remain consistent for a month or two.

First Steps Are Always the Most Difficult

Your first class or training session is often the most difficult because you may feel awkward. Everything is new and you could tire out very quickly. The second class can be equally as difficult because you may be sore from your first workout. However, by the time you finish the warm-up on day three or four, you will have worked out most of the soreness and, as long as you remain consistent, you should be through the worst of it.

Kicking Up Your Training

Once you have an understanding of the basic Krav Maga movements, it will become easier for you to put those skills together into more complex combinations. For example, rather than working only on Straight Punches, you will begin to add Hook Punches and Uppercuts into your routine. These punches will be covered in further detail in Chapter 13.

At this point the foundations of your fitness base have already been laid, so the level of intensity at which you can train will start to increase. It is safe to say that an experienced Krav Maga student will be able to train at least five days a week at sixty-plus minutes per session. This student may begin working more on refining techniques while making movements sharper, stronger, and more dynamic.

141

Whether you are a beginner or more advanced student, one thing to remember is that, no matter how fatigued you may feel while training, you should not give up. If you find yourself in a situation where you have to defend yourself, exhaustion can set in quickly and your survival may hinge on your stamina and endurance. Krav Maga practitioners keep this mentality throughout their training sessions, and students are reminded that it is possible to find strength when you feel like you may have nothing left. Sometimes strength comes directly from the mind!

The Female Warrior

The training and techniques for women are equal to those for men because Krav Maga was designed not to discriminate against students based on their sex, size, ability, or strength. Women will generally not have the same kind of upper body strength as men. They will, however, have a lower center of gravity, which means that women have a more stable foundation to maintain their balance. The unscientific observations of certain Krav Maga instructors say that women also tend to have an easier time than men when it comes to building up their physical endurance. Also, women will not (naturally) develop those massive, bulky, vein-sporting muscles that you see on some men.

Lean Muscle Without the Mass

Some women are concerned or worried about bulking up or getting too muscular when they workout. If a woman is feeling like she is getting bulky, it is usually because of dietary issues. Basically, there is too much food going in and you may begin to gain a few pounds with consistent exercise. The idea is to put on muscle while at the same time decreasing body fat percentage. Most women seek to lengthen and strengthen muscles, which is covered in Chapters 7 and 9. For more information on the dietary aspects of your training, please refer to Chapter 3.

ALERT

You can start slow, but it's not okay for you to stay at that pace for long. As your Krav Maga skills and fitness level improve, you will need to start picking up the pace. A somewhat experienced Krav Maga student (someone who has completed thirty to ninety days of regular training) should be able to increase his or her frequency and intensity of training.

Muscle tissue is highly metabolic (it uses a lot of energy and energy burns up calories) as opposed to fat, which is not metabolic at all (it is just stored energy). If you increase lean mass muscle, your body will utilize more calories all day long. This can result in the decrease of body fat as long as there are fewer or the same amount of calories coming into the body as there are going out of it.

The Effect of Hormones

It is a simple fact that women have less testosterone in their systems than men. As a result of this, women's muscles simply will not (in most cases) develop in the same way that men's muscles do. This is not to say that women do not have the same potential for strength, but simply that this strength is found in different areas (such as endurance). Generally speaking, women are considered better equipped (physiologically) for endurance activities, while men are considered to have more immediate strength. The Krav Maga self-defense system is designed so that any person, male or female, can learn to perform the techniques safely and effectively no matter what his or her size or strength might be.

13 KRAV MAGA TECHNIQUES FOR BEGINNERS

Krav Maga defines combatives as the striking techniques used both in fighting and self-defense. The majority of these exercises involve punches, kicks, and knee strikes. When it comes to keeping yourself out of harm, tools such as biting, scratching, and eye gouging are fair game in Krav Maga. This chapter will not cover elbow strikes and eye gouging, but that does not mean they are not part of the system. The techniques described are designed to cause damage to an attacker while keeping you relatively safe. Krav Maga conditioning uses these techniques to create a great workout regardless of your body shape and size.

Start with a Foundation

Your first step in Krav Maga training is learning how to stand and move properly. The way you use your feet and hold or maintain your body position affects the power of your strikes, how quickly you are able to transition from offense to defense, and the ability to maintain stability and control while moving from one skill to the next.

Neutral Stance

A neutral stance is a natural standing position. The feet should be about shoulder width apart, and your hands should be at about chin height with the elbows close to the body to protect the ribs. The hands and arms should stay relaxed and about six to eight inches away from the face. For fitness purposes, Neutral Stance is used to teach students how to rotate the body for punches and kicks without having to think about whether their right foot or left foot is forward. ■

Fighting Stance

Assuming you are right handed, begin in a neutral stance and take one natural step forward with your left foot. As you do this, the rear heel with lift off the ground slightly. Be sure the rear foot does not turn out. The toes of both feet will point forward and your body should face or be square to your opponent rather than sideways, which is commonly seen in other forms of martial arts.

The hands should be the same as in the neutral stance: at chin height with the elbows close to the body to protect the ribs. The hands and arms should stay relaxed and about six to eight inches away from the face. ▶

146

Movement

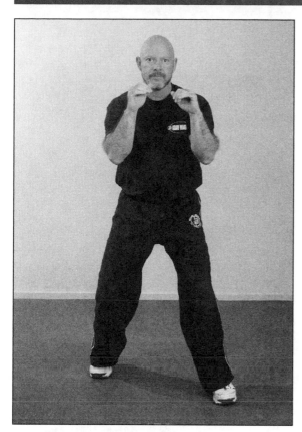

▲ FIGHTING STANCE
Stand facing forward rather than side-ways toward your opponent.

Krav Maga students need to learn how to move quickly and safely in a Fighting Stance. The basic principle is whatever direction you are moving in, that foot moves first while the other foot pushes off, finishing in a solid fighting stance. For example, begin in a Fighting Stance:

- To advance (move forward) you would move the left foot while pushing off with the right.
- To retreat (move back) you would move the right foot and push with the left.
- To move right, move the right foot and push off with the left.
- To move left, move the left foot and push off with the right.

After each movement you should land in a stable Fighting Stance. This movement is like a shuffling motion that is close to the ground. Beginners will usually hop in order to move. This is too slow and makes it hard to send a punch at the same time. Keep the feet low to the ground. One you understand basic movement, you can begin to move at different angles in diagonal lines in any direction. This method of movement allows you to keep your groin from being exposed and allows you to deliver punches while moving. ▶ *(following page)*

147

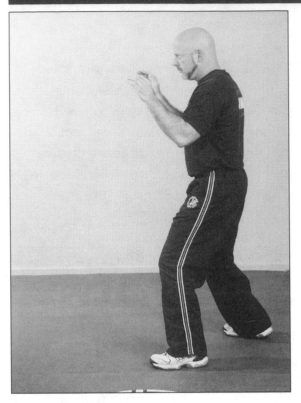

▲ ADVANCING #1
The front foot moves first.

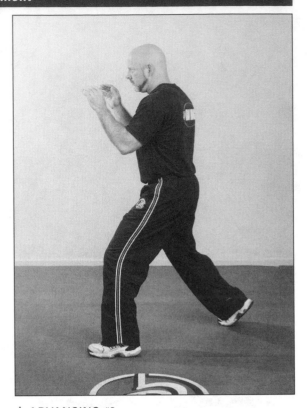

▲ ADVANCING #2
Push off with the back leg.

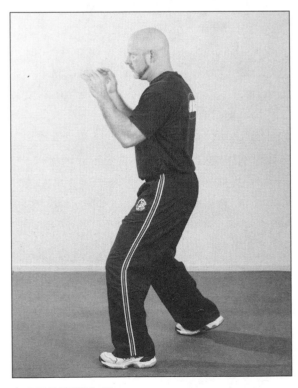

▲ ADVANCING #3
Stay low to the ground when moving your feet.

148

THE EVERYTHING KRAV MAGA FOR FITNESS BOOK

The Weapons You Cannot Drop—Hands

There is a really nice thing about human hands: Almost everyone has them and they are impossible to drop, unlike pepper spray, a knife, or any other hand-held weapon. You also can't forget them in your purse in a moment of attack. For this reason, they can be far more reliable than a hand-held weapon, especially with proper training.

In this section you are going to learn the basic mechanics of hand strikes. While there is a broad arsenal of hand strikes, this section covers just the basics. In Krav Maga fitness the most common hand strikes are left and right Straight Punches, Hook Punches, and Uppercut Punches.

Straight Punches

Straight Punches can be made with either hand. It is common in Krav Maga (and other sports) to call the left punch a "Jab" and the right punch a "Cross." Whether performing a Jab or a Cross, the basic principles of the punch are the same for either hand. In other forms of martial arts and fighting, the Jab is used as either a distraction punch (used in a quick tapping motion that does not have a lot of power behind it), or it is used to determine the distance between you and an opponent. In Krav Maga, students are taught to make every attack count. So a left Jab in Krav Maga is meant to do damage, not just distract or disturb your opponent. Keep this in mind during your training sessions.

A Straight Punch is a medium-range weapon, so be sure you are standing with enough distance from your target to extend your punch all the way out without jamming yourself. You should be a little more than one arms length from the target.

When performing a Straight Punch, as the hand travels forward it's important to keep the elbow down as long as possible. This ensures the punch travels in one straight line, which is the shortest distance to the target. It also makes a smaller, less detectable movement and keeps the ribs protected for a longer period of time while delivering the strike. As you send the punch, the shoulder and hip rotate forward adding reach and power to the punch. ▼

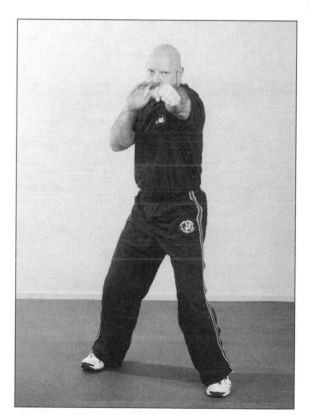

▲ LEFT STRAIGHT PUNCH
Send the left hand out and back without dropping the opposite hand.

149

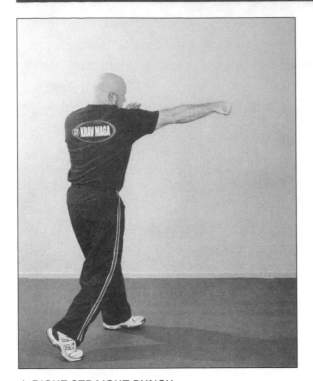

▲ RIGHT STRAIGHT PUNCH
*Bring the right side of the body for-
ward when delivering a right cross.*

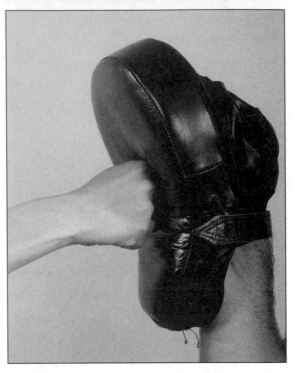

▲ HOW TO HIT
Make contact with the first two knuckles.

As contact is made, the wrist should rotate 45 degrees to add power. Contact is made with the first two knuckles, keeping the wrist straight. Recoil the hand quickly back to its starting position following the same path it was delivered on. Once you are comfortable with this movement you can tuck the chin and rotate the shoulder on the punching side up to protect the jaw.

SAFETY

The left Jab is usually not going to feel as strong as the right Cross. This is because the right Cross has a further distance to travel before making contact, and during that time it is able to gain velocity. You should still train with the purpose of making your left punch just as strong as your right punch.

Begin in a Fighting Stance, and as the left hand moves forward into the punch, use the legs by pushing off the ground and rotate the left shoulder and hip forward. Extend the punch all the way out and recoil back to your starting position. Again, the hand rotates about 45 degrees upon impact.

150

One last thing to think about when sending a punch (or any attack) is to try to send your punch through the pad rather than tapping the surface of the pad. In order to do this well you have to have your weight behind your punch at the point of impact. It will make your punch have a great deal of power.

Holding the Focus Mitts

The pad holder (this is your partner) should hold the pads in front of her shoulders and have them facing the puncher (you). The puncher will send the left punch to the pad holder's left hand and the right punch to the pad holder's right hand. As the punch is just about to make contact the pad holder should catch the punch so there is a little bit of resistance for the puncher. Otherwise the pads would fly back as contact is made. Your partner should be in a solid stance and use his or her legs and abs to absorb the impact.

If you are acting as the pad holder, be sure that you are not slamming down onto your partner's hands when he punches! This can hurt the puncher's wrist.

It takes practice to hold the pads just as it takes practice to learn to punch. Use the time you are holding the pads to learn to read what the punches look like when being delivered toward you. It's a great visual drill and can teach you a lot about fighting. ▼

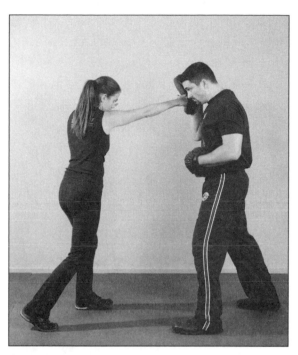

▲ HOLDING THE FOCUS MITTS
Holding mitts properly takes practice.

151

Advancing Straight Punches

A Straight Punch can be made with an advance in order to cover distance while you punch. This punch is done with a significant amount of distance between you and your target so you have the space to move forward into the attack. If you think about a sparring situation, the two fighters do not stand one arm's distance from each other the whole time. They maintain a certain amount of distance then burst in and send a punch or combination of punches. This is the idea of advancing in.

As you send your left Jab forward, immediately burst forward with an advance, pushing off with the rear foot and moving the forward foot. As the punch lands, the rear foot should close the distance. In most cases, the advance should be on a slight diagonal to keep you away from the opponent's range of attacks. This technique is the same for punching with the rear hand or advancing into a left-right combination. Usually you would not advance in, deliver one punch, and then just stay there. You should either follow up with more punches or retreat out. ▶

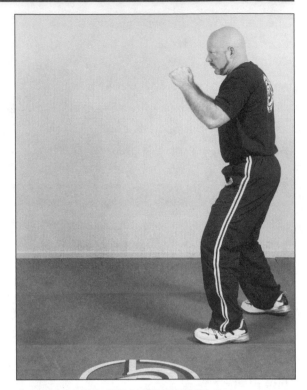

▲ ADVANCING STRAIGHT PUNCH #1
Start in a Fighting Stance.

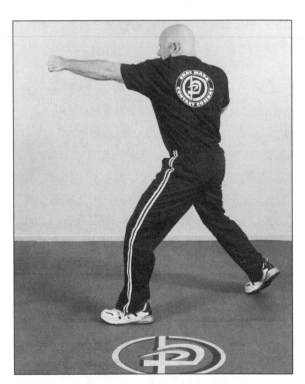

▲ ADVANCING STRAIGHT PUNCH #2
Move the left hand and left foot forward into the attack.

152

THE EVERYTHING KRAV MAGA FOR FITNESS BOOK

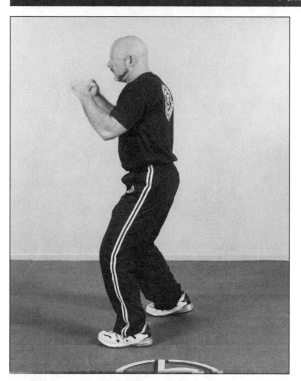

▲ ADVANCING STRAIGHT PUNCH #3
End in a solid Fighting Stance.

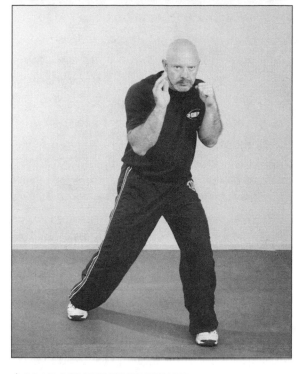

▲ LOAD FOR THE HOOK PUNCH
Load your weight on the left leg.

Hook Punches

A Hook Punch is usually used when the opponent is fairly close. The target of a Hook Punch is the side of the opponent's face or body, which means the strike will be "hooking" in from the side. Rather than punching straight ahead, the elbow bends and the punch is delivered around the opponent's hands and arms.

To begin the punch, bring the elbow up so the arm is parallel to the floor. The elbow should remain bent throughout the punch. The shoulder and hip rotate forward and in, adding weight and power behind the punch. When making contact, the wrist should rotate 45 degrees, just as a Straight Punch. Be sure your wrist is straight upon impact. Any bend in the wrist can cause a wrist injury. ▶

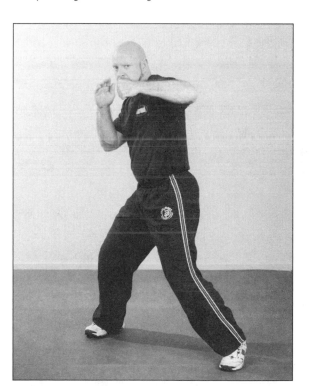

▲ HOOK PUNCH
Then unwind your weight into your punch.

153

The Hook Punch can be delivered to the face or the body, and the elbow determines the height of the punch. So if you are delivering a Hook to the body, the elbow does not need to come up as high. Either way, you want to have your weight into the punch upon contact.

There are two ways to recoil from the Hook Punch. You can either drop the elbow down and bring the hand back up to the guard position, which tends to be the faster of the two, or you can recoil the punch back in the same path it was sent on. When working to a heavy bag the latter is usually the best choice. Either way is acceptable.

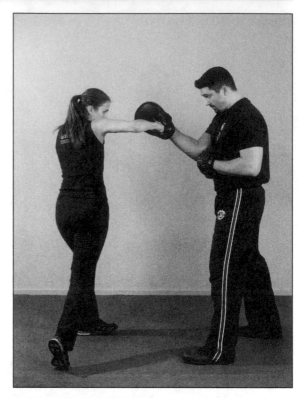

▲ HOOK PUNCH TO MITT
Be sure to make contact with the first two knuckles.

The left Hook may not feel as strong as the right Hook. Try to pivot your left foot slightly when sending the left Hook, which you may find helpful in getting your weight behind your punch. Beginners have a tendency to tighten up their entire body when learning to punch and move their arm and body as one unit. The arms and body should move independently but connected to each other. If you feel this is the case, slow down and focus on staying relaxed.

Holding the focus mitts for this punch: When holding the mitts, the pad should be held at the midline of the puncher's body. Be sure to angle the pad slightly outward. If the surface is perpendicular to the puncher it can hurt his or her wrist. ▶

154

Uppercut Punches

Uppercut and Hook Punches can be thought of as the same punch delivered at different angles. Whereas for a Hook Punch the body moves forward and in, the Uppercut rotates the body and moves it forward and upward.

As the Uppercut Punch begins there is a slight bend in the knees and waist. This drops you below the target slightly. As the punch develops, the hand moves out and up as the same side shoulder rotates in and up. The elbow should stay close to the body to protect the ribs.

As the punch moves toward the target, drive up with the legs to add power. When making contact, the palm of the hand should be facing toward you with the elbow under the fist. Recoil the punch back in the same path it was sent on. This punch is similar to the action of a piston.

SAFETY

Beware! Your hand should not drop down to the waist in order to deliver the punch upward. This exposes the side of the head for an attack, so as you drop down, keep your hands up. Your punch may not feel as strong, but the risk of dropping your hand is much greater than the reward of a stronger punch.

Be sure the punch is not coming back toward your face. If you are not punching to a target it is hard to see if this is happening. Remember, your target is out in front of you, so your punch has to move forward and up rather than back toward your face. Again, this is easier to feel when working to a focus mitt. If your punch feels like it is sliding off the pad, slow down and pay attention to the angle you are sending the punch.

Holding the focus mitts for this punch: For the Uppercut the pad should be held at the height of the puncher's chin. The pad should not be facing the floor. It should be angled slightly forward to the puncher so the punch can be delivered forward and up. ▼

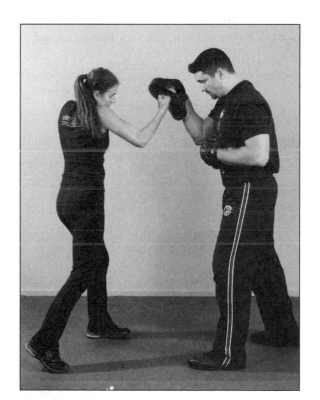

▲ UPPERCUT TO MITT
The same punch is done whether making contact to a mitt or not.

155

CHAPTER 13   KRAV MAGA TECHNIQUES FOR BEGINNERS

Combinations

Once you feel comfortable with the basic punches you can begin to work on combinations of punches. A combination is a series of punches. What distinguishes a combination is as you recoil one punch the next punch is beginning to develop. Think of it as punches passing each other in front of you rather than sending one punch, stopping, and then throwing another punch.

SAFETY

Keep in mind that, when working to a heavy bag, you do not have a correct target for an Uppercut. It is not recommended to practice Uppercuts to the bag. If you put an Uppercut into a combination while working on the heavy bag, have the back of your hand slide up along the bag to simulate the punch.

The most basic combination is a left-right punch combo. As you send the left punch, the right hand is ready to follow. When the left hand comes back, the right hand is delivered. The emphasis should be placed on driving with the legs and hip in order to generate power behind both punches. Once you are comfortable with that, try adding a left Hook off the right Cross. Again, emphasize shifting your weight from your left to your right as you send the left Hook by driving with the legs and hips.

The last addition is the right Uppercut. From the left Hook, drop down slightly and drive your weight forward and up into your right Uppercut. Recoil your hand back to your face and move your feet as your would in a fight.

Wearing Hand Wraps

You should wear hand wraps when training on the heavy bag or to focus mitts. When learning how to punch, the position of the wrist is not always straight as it should be. Wearing hand wraps can help to stabilize the wrist and avoid any wrist injuries. Hand wraps also provide hand support for the delicate joints in the hand.

In the beginning you may find that your hands are a little sore from punching. You have muscles and tendons in your hands that need to be strengthened and adapt to the impact required with punching. If you are not wearing gloves while punching, hand wraps protect the skin of your knuckles from getting torn up. It may be a wise choice to purchase a pair of gloves to protect the hands and wrists from overuse injuries.

How to Wrap Your Hands

Try to purchase a pair of wraps that are fairly long and have some stretch to them. This will make it easier to wrap and will be more comfortable for the hand. The idea is to have wrist support, hand support, and coverage of the knuckles. As you wrap your hand, keep your hand open and fingers spread.

ESSENTIAL

If there is any length of wrap left over, use it for extra wrist support. If your hand begins to fall asleep, you may have wrapped it too tight. Your wraps should feel supportive without cutting off circulation to your hands.

Begin by anchoring the loop around the thumb and pull the wrap tight toward the pinky side of the wrist. Wrap it around the wrist a couple of times so it feels snug. From the thumb side of the wrist, loop the wrap though each finger and back around the wrist one at a time, always coming back to the thumb side as an anchor. Once you have gone through each finger, finishing on the outside of the pinky, figure-8 the wrap from the palm of the hand to the wrist until the wrap looks clean and feels snug.

14 BUILDING ON TECHNIQUE

You now have a foundation for striking with your hands. When delivering the punches in the preceding chapter you had a stable foundation because both feet were on the ground when you made contact. This in not the case when using your feet or your knees to strike. In order to kick or deliver a knee strike, you will have to be on one leg for a brief period of time. This requires you to have a certain amount of stability and balance to deliver a solid strike to a target.

159

Long-Range Weapons—Kicks

Kicks are more powerful than punches. Why? First of all, your legs are much stronger than your arms. They have been holding you up since the day you learned to walk and they carry your weight around all day long. Your legs are also longer than your arms, meaning kicks will give you a much greater reach advantage (which might even your odds against an opponent with longer arms who is untrained in using or defending against kicks). Legs are also harder to see coming than a punch.

Your legs are also far more crucial to your ability to maintain balance than are your hands and arms. Anytime you kick to targets that are above waist level you risk losing your balance. Therefore, Krav Maga often stresses kicking to vulnerable targets located in the lower areas of the body—such as the legs, knees, and groin. However, remember that when you are kicking you are also standing on one leg, even if only for a brief moment. This means you are temporarily unstable (compared to the stability of having both your feet on the ground).

Front Kicks

In Krav Maga there are two basic Front Kicks. The first is a kick to the groin using the instep or shin, and the second is a kick to a vertical target, which acts more like a punch with the ball of your foot toward your opponents midsection.

In sport fighting, such as mixed martial arts, kicking to the groin is not allowed. The reason these kicks are illegal is because a groin kick is hard to see coming, therefore it is very challenging to defend against. Also, when a groin kick lands correctly it is very damaging and can end the fight! This is the very reason it is allowed and encouraged in the Krav Maga training system. When it comes to self-defense, the Front Kick to the groin is a highly effective tool.

A Front Kick is a swinging of the leg combined with an opening and closing of the knee. Krav Maga emphasizes not just kicking to your target but kicking through the target. Remember, you want your foot to travel further than the contact point, which is why this kick may look like a high kick when performing it without making contact. Once you are comfortable kicking with the rear leg, practice kicking with the front leg. Kicking to the groin with the forward leg may feel less powerful, but it is faster and sneakier. Remember that you make contact with this kick with either the area of the foot where you would tie your shoes or with your shin.

An additional Front Kick used in Krav Maga is a Front Kick with the ball of the foot. This kick is delivered to the midsection or chest. In order to make contact with the ball of your foot you need to pull your toes upward to the top of your shoes to expose the ball of the foot. If you are not sure, kick the ground with the ball of your foot a few times to understand the striking surface. The ball of the foot is very bony, and if this kick is delivered appropriately it can penetrate you opponent's body and do a great deal of damage.

This kick can be practiced without making contact to a pad, but to feel the effectiveness of the kick it should be executed to a heavy bag. This kick is considered a long-range weapon, so be sure you have enough distance between you and the bag. ▼▶

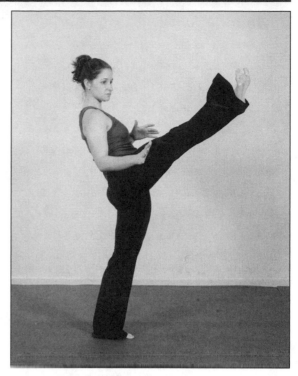

▲ FRONT KICK STEP 2
As the hip of the kicking leg comes forward the knee extends out and recoils back, placing the foot back in its original fighting stance position.

Keep your hands up as you deliver the kick so you are in a position to defend yourself against a possible attack or counter-attack to your head. Once you are more experienced with kicks, it is not necessary to always land back in your Fighting Stance. You may find that you land in a Neutral Stance or your opposite Fighting Stance, where what was your back foot is now forward. Either way, after delivering a strong kick you should be in control and able to plant the kicking foot wherever it is needed.

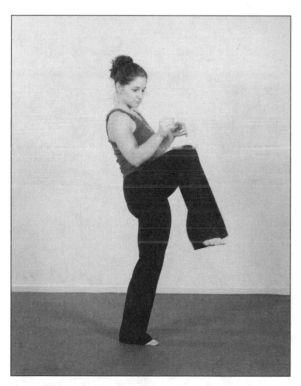

▲ FRONT KICK STEP 1
From a Fighting Stance, swing the rear leg forward with the knee bent.

161

Round Kicks

Just as a Hook Punch (Chapter 13, page 153) and an Uppercut Punch (Chapter 13, page 155) are the same punch on different planes, the same holds true for a Front Kick versus a Round Kick. A Round Kick is essentially a Front Kick turned over on its side. The striking surface for a round kick is the same as a Front Kick—the area of the shoelaces or the shin. You can use a Round Kick to strike the knee, the leg, the ribs, or even the head. Although Krav Maga self-defense does not emphasize kicks to the head because they are hard to make effective, there is a place for them in fitness training because they foster balance, flexibility, and control.

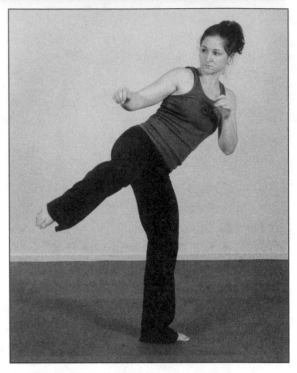

▲ ROUND KICK, NO CONTACT STEP 1
Begin with your left base foot turned out so your heel is pointed toward the direction you are kicking.

Round Kick Without Making Contact

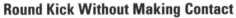

This kick is much less complex due to the fact that since you are not striking anything you do not have to think about angles of contact. When performing a Round Kick without a bag or pad, you cannot put nearly as much weight into your kick because you have nothing for your leg to strike. Practicing this kick is great for balance and stability as well as flexibility and mobility of the hips.

Begin with your left foot, which is your base foot, turned out at about 45 degrees. Next, pick the right knee up, extend the leg out and back, then lightly place the right foot on the floor. ▶

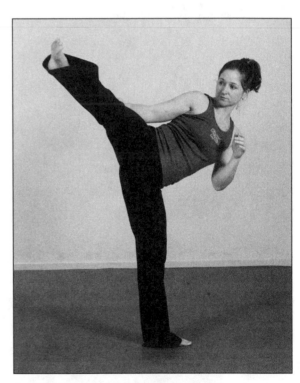

▲ ROUND KICK, NO CONTACT STEP 2
Pick the right knee up, extend the leg out and back, then lightly place the right foot on the floor and repeat.

162

Round Kick to a Heavy Bag

A Round Kick to a Heavy Bag takes practice. Take your time, be patient, and don't try to kick the bag with full speed. Learn the movement first and it will begin to become more powerful as your technique improves.

When you first learn a Round Kick, begin in a Neutral Stance. Pick the right knee up and roll the right hip over while pivoting on the base foot. The knee will open to send the kick and close to recoil the kick, just as it does for a Front Kick. As you recoil, be sure the base foot pivots back to where it started.

You may place the kicking leg in either a Fighting Stance or a Neutral Stance. The most important part is that you know where you want to place the leg and you are able to place it there in a controlled manner.▼ (*and following page*)

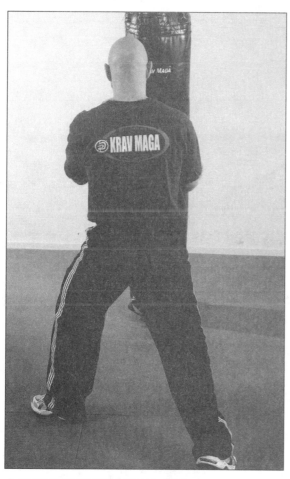

▲ ROUND KICK TO A HEAVY BAG #1
Begin in a Neutral Stance and take a slight step in the direction you are going to kick.

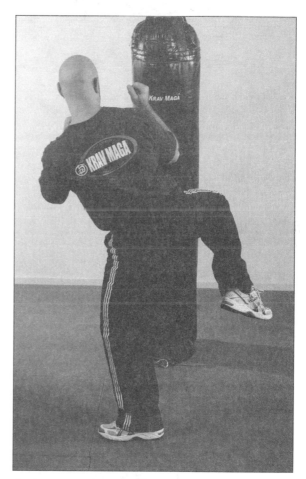

▲ ROUND KICK TO A HEAVY BAG #2
Pick up the knee of the kicking leg.

163

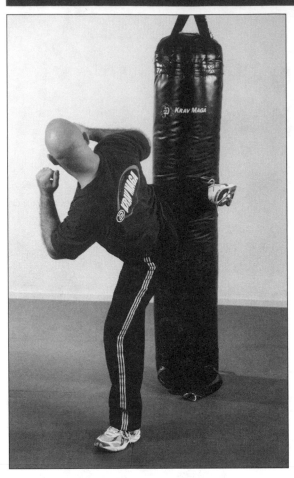

Another common problem with the Round Kick is not getting the hip to roll over or turn on its side. This problem can often be fixed by pivoting the foot. Try facing the bag, then send a right kick and pause with your shin on the bag. Observe that your right hip should be directly on top of the left hip. Try holding this position for a count of five or until you feel solid in that position. Practice this kick and hold it a few times, then see if you can apply that motion into your kick.

▲ ROUND KICK TO A HEAVY BAG #3
Pivot the base foot, turn the leg on its side, and make contact with the shin.

A common problem in executing a Round Kick is the base foot not pivoting enough or at all. The reason for pivoting this foot is to allow the hips to move in the direction the kick is going. Many students try to pivot on a flat foot, or lift the ball of their foot and do not pivot at all. This can cause undue torque and stress to the knee. Be sure when you pivot that you are turning on the ball of the foot so that the heel comes almost completely forward. It may help to take the weight off the foot, almost like you are jumping.

Knee Strikes

The Knee Strike is a weapon that is used when you are very close to your opponent. If you have ever seen a mixed martial arts fight, fighters in close to each other try to send Knee Strikes to the body in many angles and directions. For the purpose of basic fitness this section will go over Knee Strikes that travels forward and upward.

Knee Strike to a Heavy Bag

When delivering a Knee Strike to a Heavy Bag, place one hand on each side of the bag. Bring the knee up and at the same time move your hips forward and up to generate power. Lightly touch the knee to the bag, then place the foot back down and repeat. ■

Knee Strike Without Making Contact

When practicing Knee Strikes Without Making Contact, imagine you are grabbing the shoulder and back of your opponent's arm. As your knee travels upward, you pull your hands down toward your knee as if you were pulling your opponent's upper body down into your knee. The two forces moving toward each other will have a much greater impact upon collision than if only one force was moving. ▶

▲ KNEE STRIKE WITHOUT MAKING CONTACT
Keep your heel close to your buttocks in order to make the knee a sharp surface that can penetrate a target.

165

Side Kicks

A Side Kick is different than a Front Kick or Round Kick because it's similar to a stomping kick. It is the same movement you would use to stomp on an aluminum can to crush it, but the stomp is done out to the side. This kick is usually delivered to the midsection but can also be done to the knee.

When working to a heavy bag you need to have a significant amount of distance between you and the bag. Start by standing sideways to the bag. Bring the knee that is closest to the bag up in front of your body in a chambered position, with the foot raised and the knee bent high. Extend your kicking leg and hips out toward the target while pivoting your base foot so that your heel turns toward the target. You should make contact with the bottom of your heel with your foot parallel to the floor. Recoil by bringing your foot and knee back toward you, then return it to the floor. ▶

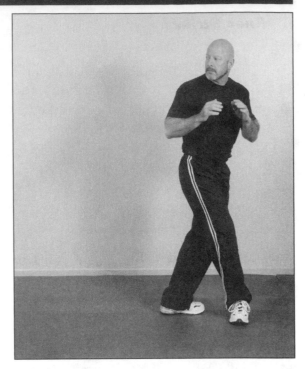

▲ SIDE KICK #1
Turn the heel of the base foot toward the target.

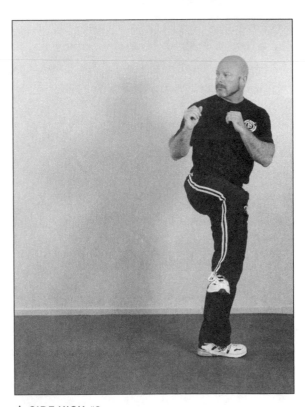

▲ SIDE KICK #2
Bring the knee up to load the kick.

166

Don't leave your leg hanging out there once you've delivered a sidekick. Pull it back in the opposite direction that you delivered. You want to be on one leg for as short a time as possible.

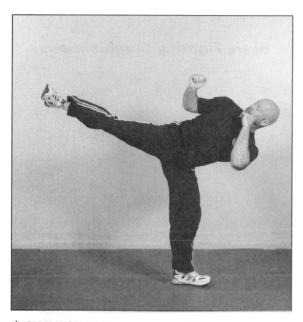

▲ SIDE KICK #3
Extend the leg out, making contact with the heel of the foot.

If it is hard for you to lift the knee and pivot the base foot, you may want to try stepping into your Side Kick. You will need a little more distance for this Side Kick because you are stepping in toward the bag. When standing sideways to the bag, step behind the kicking leg. When you take this step, be sure you place the foot with the heel pointed toward the bag, chamber your knee, and send the Side Kick the same way as above.

Side Kick Without Making Contact

Performing a Side Kick that does not make contact requires the same movements as if you were making contact to a target. One thing you need to be aware of is not to hyperextend the knee upon the extension of the kick. Begin slowly and control the motion out and back with the leg. Once this feels stable you can then begin to kick with more intent. Keep in mind that you do not put as much force into attacks that do not have a bag or pad to make contact with. ■

167

Building Combinations

Once you are comfortable with all of the combatives you have learned thus far you should begin practicing your efficiency at delivering them in combinations of well-controlled flurries. Combinations should not be wild. They are clean, controlled sequences of various striking techniques that are delivered in a rapid and overlapping succession to one or more targets on your opponent(s). This requires much more work out of you than you have experienced while practicing multiple solo combatives. In the long run, however, it makes for a much better offense than simply practicing one combative at a time.

Training to deliver effective strike combinations will require you to develop good balance, cultivate your skill at shifting your weight properly, and will test your ability to maintain a good Fighting Stance while your entire body is in motion (both the upper and lower half).

Punch-Kick Combinations

When putting combinations together, as one strike comes back the other strike begins to develop. The momentum of one attack can help increase the power of the next attack. In a Krav Maga conditioning program there are four basic fighting combinations that are commonly practiced and trained on a heavy bag. The number indicates how many alternating punches are going to be delivered, leading with a Jab and ending with the opposite leg Round Kick to finish the combination.

For instance, Basic #3 would be three punches, left-right-left, followed up with the opposite leg kick. Since the last punch was a left punch, you would finish with a right leg Round Kick.

Basic Fighting Combinations

These combinations can only be practiced with a heavy bag because of how the weight and force is transferred while performing the combinations. The basic four fighting combinations are as follows:

- Basic #1 = left punch, right round kick
- Basic #2 = left-right punch, left round kick
- Basic #3 = left-right-left punch, right round kick
- Basic #4 = left-right-left-right punch, left round kick

Once you have mastered these combinations with Straight Punches (Chapter 13, page 149), every time you have a third punch (as in combinations 3 and 4) you can change that punch to a Hook Punch.

Delivering a Round Kick from the forward leg is a more advanced kick because you need to understand how to keep enough distance between you and the bag in order to have enough space to develop the kick. It's also a weaker kick so it does not feel as satisfying as kicking with the back leg. Knowing this you should understand that basic fighting combos 2 and 4 will feel more challenging to make strong and solid to the bag since they both end with a forward leg Round Kick. Practice combinations 1 and 3 until you feel like you have mastered those before moving on to combinations 2 and 4.

Knocked Down? Get Up Again

Just because you're down doesn't necessarily mean that you have to be out. While you'd prefer not to get knocked down in a fight, in Krav Maga you must train for every possible scenario. Therefore, you must be prepared even for the situations that you would normally try to avoid.

Over the last decade, the world of mixed martial arts fighting has raised awareness about the importance of being able to fight effectively from the ground. Not being prepared for the moment when you find yourself on your back could put you in a situation that quickly goes from bad to worse.

Defending from the Ground

While Krav Maga is usually a standing/striking system, it does recognize that fights very often go to the ground. One of the reasons Krav Maga emphasizse a balanced Fighting Stance is to reduce the likelihood of you falling or getting taken to the ground. Krav Maga students are, however, trained to deal with this situation. If you end up on the ground, you should place yourself on your back or on your side and use your legs as weapons to keep your opponent away from you.

Striking Back Even When You're Down

What if there is no time to get back up? What if you are down and your attacker is coming at you? Have you ever heard the saying that the best defense is a good offense? Your opponent is going to try to take advantage of what he views as a vulnerable position for you. But for your opponent, this would be a misconception at best and an underestimation at worst. There are a number of methods for striking at your opponent from a position on the ground that can give you an opportunity to even the playing field or simply give you the time and opening necessary to regain your footing. The recommended striking method when on the ground is the Side Kick, although other strikes can work well, too.

169

Remember that "down" does not have to translate into "out," not in combat and certainly not in Krav Maga. As you begin training, you need to cultivate the thought that there is no such thing as "out" for you. As long as you have a limb that works and breath in your lungs, you are not and will not be defeated.

Side Kick from the Ground

The Side Kick from the side position is a great way to strengthen the side of the waist and core, and it also strengthens the hips, particularly the gluteus muscles. Begin on the ground on your side so you are on your elbow, hip, and base leg. Keep your other hand up in front of your face. The top leg is chambered and ready to kick. As you extend the leg out, your hips will lift and move toward the target. The same rules apply for Side Kicks on the ground as they do for standing. Make contact with the heel and recoil back to your starting position.

If you do not have a heavy bag, you can do any of these kicks without making contact. Just be sure you do not hyperextend the knee when kicking out. Stay in control of your kick and focus on balance and coordination of the technique. ▶

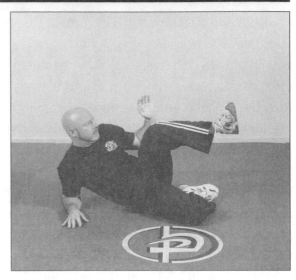

▲ SIDE KICK FROM THE GROUND #1
Start on the forearm and hip.

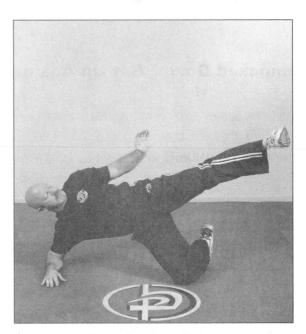

▲ SIDE KICK FROM THE GROUND #2
Extend the leg out, lifting the hips off the ground and toward the target.

Shadowboxing Versus Hitting a Target

Shadowboxing is simply the act of throwing combatives at the air, at your shadow on the wall, or at your own reflection. You are attacking and defending against an imaginary opponent. Shadowboxing allows you to practice all the combatives, as well as moving in, out, and around while maintaining a good Fighting Stance.

Shadowboxing develops the muscles that are used to recoil a strike, since it is your own body (not momentum) that stops the motion and draws your weapons back to a comfortable Fighting Stance. It also allows you to move more freely, simulating another potential reality of a fight. Shadowboxing also allows some students, especially those who are not yet used to a high level of impact, to keep working out without putting too much stress on their joints.

Hitting a Target

Shadowboxing allows you to strike without the concern of a target, but you can't shadowbox forever. Hitting a target presents its own set of realities. You have to hold your fist correctly to avoid injury to your hand. Also, you will begin to develop additional elements of your striking game. As you begin striking an actual target, whether it be focus mitts or a heavy bag, you will develop the following physical attributes and skills:

- Accuracy
- Contact/impact
- Movement
- Range
- Power

Helpful Hints for the Beginning Striker and Kicker

For those of you who may be throwing punches and kicks for the first time in your lives, please remember a few simple things to keep your introduction to Krav Maga techniques as safe and injury free as possible. Remember to start off gradually, because getting injured is counterproductive to both your personal fitness and Krav Maga goals. You can't train at 100 percent if you are hurt. A few other points to keep in mind:

- Start out your punch routines with shadowboxing.
- Once you feel comfortable with the technique and your performance, make light contact to a flexible target such as a striking shield or focus mitts.
- Slowly work your way up to the heavy bag.
- Pay attention to the point of contact, making sure that your range is good and that you are not going to injure yourself once you begin making contact to a target.

ESSENTIAL

When delivering a strike, you want to make sure that you make contact at the sweet spot. This means that you are at the proper distance from your target (not coming up short or jamming your attack) and are making contact at the most powerful point of your attack.

It simply can't be stressed enough—do not just let your hands fly when you are throwing punches at a target. This is imperative! Remember the proper punching technique and be aware that the position of your hand and points of contact in these punches are a certain way for a very good reason: to prevent you from breaking your hands! Don't get lazy with the form of your punches. You might end up paying for your laziness with a sprained or broken hand or wrist.

15 SKILL-RELATED COMPONENTS

There are a number of essential skills within a well-balanced Krav Maga fitness program that you will need to incorporate into your training and practice. These skills—balance, speed, coordination, power, agility, and reaction time—are all universally important components of almost any athletic activity. The well-rounded professional athlete maintains a high level of proficiency in all of these skills. This proficiency of skill-related components is why a gymnast is able to pick up an activity such as ice-skating much faster than an individual without any prior skill-related training.

Importance of Skill-Related Components

When analyzing the demands of any sport, it is important to examine the necessary skills involved within the movements of that particular sport. Take a look at tennis. The demands of tennis are that players must be fast to get to the ball and react quickly as well as accurately to whatever their opponent does. The tennis player needs to have the ability to switch directions and angles in an instant. In order to switch directions rapidly, she will need to have a certain amount of balance. In order to hit a tennis ball with sufficient accuracy, a tennis player needs to coordinate and control her body movements in a particularly efficient fashion. Lastly, the tennis athlete needs to have a certain amount of muscular power in order to allow her to project the ball with enough force to challenge the opposing player.

By practicing these skill-related elements, you will have the ability to increase your performance in any sport or activity. This is why Krav Maga fitness training programs include exercises that encompass and enforce all of these skills as equally as possible. This way you will train to become a more skilled fighter whether you are in the training room or on the street.

Agility

The standard definition of agility is the ability to change directions quickly. Agility is an integral component in Krav Maga. Most sports require players to stop and start their movements at the drop of a hat. Even dancers must train for agility.

> **ESSENTIAL**
>
> You will grow stronger through strength and functional training exercises, faster through the practice of speed training and speed drills, more coordinated through functional training exercises where the limbs have to move correctly with each other, and create a better center of balance through the practice of balancing drills, all the while becoming a more well-rounded athlete.

Take soccer, for example. The players run up and down the field with little to no rest throughout the game. They could be running in one direction and in an instant have to decelerate, stabilize the momentum of their bodyweight, coordinate the shift of that weight, create enough momentum to start moving that weight in a new direction, and accelerate as quickly as possible. This is why agility is dependent on strength, speed, coordination, and dynamic balance. If you can train for all of these elements, you will experience an improvement in your agility. The more you practice agility, and the components found within agility, the more your agility will improve.

Applying Agility to Krav Maga

Agility is beneficial to any fighter, whether in Krav Maga or some other discipline. If you look at the movements involved in a sparring match, you will see that the fighters are constantly moving their feet in a myriad of directions: left, right, forward, back, in, and out. Clean and stable footwork, as well as the ability to make quick adjustments of your body (as a whole or in parts), are crucial elements in professional fighting.

FACT

It is a good idea for fighters to train regularly at becoming agile in a small space. The best way to do this is to train and spar in a small space. You may want to perform drills, such as moving quickly from side to side over a line on the floor, or move forward and back by pushing off with one foot at a time (such as you learned while advancing and retreating).

Fighters have to be able to move in an infinite amount of angles (and do it within a finite amount of space) without letting their feet slip, turning their backs to their opponents, or letting their defensive posture drop. Even though fighters are not running up and down a soccer field or basketball court, they are still required to change directions very quickly, but they have to do so in a far smaller area and a more confined space, such as within the ropes of a boxing ring or the octagonal-shaped cages used in the Ultimate Fighting Championship (UFC) and other MMA/NHB fighting arenas.

Lateral Movement with a Line Drill

This is a good exercise to improve your agility. Stand on one side of a line (just run a piece of tape down the floor that is a foot or more in length) and quickly jump or hop with both feet from one side to the other. Once you get going, work on becoming as light on your feet as possible. Start increasing your speed as you begin to become more accustomed to the rhythm of the exercise.

SAFETY

It's easy to roll an ankle when you are working on lateral movement. Be aware of how you push off your foot when moving from side to side. Start slowly and begin to increase your speed as you become more stable with the movements.

Once you find a comfortable rhythm, you should start performing this exercise for time, such as hopping back and forth without rest for twenty to thirty seconds. If you don't feel ready for a timed version of this drill, you may want to start out by just doing this for a certain number of repetitions, such as doing ten to twenty hops (over and back again should equal one repetition).

For added difficulty, you can perform this lateral movement with a line drill by hopping back and forth on only one foot at a time. The same rules apply as when you perform this exercise with both legs. Try staying as close to the line as possible without touching it. This helps increase lower leg strength and stability in the ankles. ■

CHAPTER 15 SKILL-RELATED COMPONENTS

Lateral Movement with Cones Drill

Place two cones on the ground, about three to four feet apart. Start inside the cones and, as quickly as possible, move laterally (sideways) back and forth as fast as you can, touching each cone before moving to the next. Repeat this exercise for a total of ten repetitions (from one cone to the other and back is one repetition).

ESSENTIAL

Cones are a suggestion for this drill, not a requirement. Anything that will stay where you put it and mark the necessary spots on the ground will suffice. For example, a pair of hand weights, a couple of water bottles, some bricks, empty coffee cans—any of these would do the job. Not having cones is no reason to not perform this exercise drill.

Remember, your focus needs to be on agility. With that in mind, you are going to want to pay close attention to quickly switching your direction. Do this by pushing off with your outside leg. Just as with the line version of this drill, you can also do this exercise for time, again twenty- to thirty-second intervals. ∎

Speed

Speed is the ability to perform a movement within a short period of time. Most sports have some sort of speed component. The team or individual who is the fastest is usually the one who scores more points/goals/runs. Speed is important in Krav Maga for a few reasons. First, in order to defend yourself from an attacker you have to make your defense in a very short period of time. The slower you are at defending yourself, the more time your attacker has to attack and control you. As soon as the attacker sees that you are planning on making a defense, he can prepare, and then it may end up being a fight that is decided by which of you is the stronger rather than quicker. More often than not, the fighter who is the stronger will win.

The thing that makes Krav Maga self-defense so effective is that you, the practitioner, are trained to not only defend against and respond to a strong attacker with speed, but not to stop responding until the situation has been neutralized or you are able to get away from it safely. Not only is it important to defend with speed, but you also want to counterattack with speed as well. The faster you can send punches and knees, the harder it will be for your opponent to see them coming.

The same holds true for the martial arts that have been adapted into sports. When MMA fighters are sparring, a punch that is telegraphed or thrown too slowly is easy to see coming and will be easy to defend against. The same is true for kicks and knees, so it's important to train the muscles in your upper and lower body to move the necessary limbs in a short period of time.

Training for Increased Speed

It is possible to increase your speed by working on your punches and kicks while focusing on making them faster. What you must realize is that when there is an increase in speed there can be a loss of force behind your attacks, which can translate into a lack of power. If you are concentrating purely on increasing your speed, this may not be such a problem. If you want to increase your striking power, however, which should be a goal in your Krav Maga training, compromising the force of your attacks for the sake of increasing your speed may not be the best of ideas. A lack of power behind your strikes will result in your inflicting less damage to someone who may be trying to hurt you.

You can take just about any skill and work on making it faster. If you want to make your left-right punch combinations faster, you should work on that combination while focusing on speed and technique. You can increase the number of punches you throw in rapid succession in order to challenge yourself, repeating six alternating straight punches and doing so over and over with the intention of making them as fast as possible without neglecting proper technique!

ALERT

An increase in the speed at which you perform a technique (especially kicks), if done improperly, can lead to joint damage or other injuries. For example, when many beginners start performing a Round Kick with increased speed, they often neglect the positioning of their base foot. This improper technique can lead to a torque of the hip joint in the base leg that can cause joint damage.

You may notice that your legs or feet are not moving as fast as you'd like them to. You can work on developing speed in your lower body by performing the drills listed above for agility, or by employing the exercises that are listed in the next section.

177

High Knees Drill

This purpose behind High Knees is to get your legs moving faster. This exercise is done as though you are running, except there should be little to no forward travel or momentum. While running in place, focus on picking your knee up as fast as you can while remaining light on your feet. If you are heavy on your feet, it will usually cause your movements to be slow and your attacks to be telegraphed. Do not forget to keep your arms moving as well. A rapid arm swing can cause your legs to react faster. Draw your navel in by keeping your abs tight and tipping your torso forward just slightly. This exercise should be done for time not repetitions. Performing this exercise for anywhere from ten to thirty seconds is sufficient enough for results. It will increase your heart rate significantly, so this can also be done as an interval. ■

ESSENTIAL

Sprinting is also a great way to train your legs for speed and power. Determine a distance and clearly mark the beginning and end points. Try getting from one point to the other as fast as you can. Time yourself with a stopwatch, record your times, then repeat it again the next week and see if you can beat the previous times.

A Loss of Stability

There comes a point in speed training where you will actually begin to lose the stability of the skill being performed. For example, say you are trying to make your Round Kicks faster and you choose to do a speed drill in which you are standing in front of a heavy bag with your focus being to kick the bag as fast as you can five times. If your only goal is to make your five kicks faster, then at some point you are going to lose all of the other components that go into the Round Kick. Too much speed can result in a lack of some very crucial skills, such as instability in your dynamic balance, incorrect or non-existent rotation/pivoting of your base foot, misaligned rotations of your pelvis, and the accuracy in making contact with a target. When all of these elements are thrown out for the sake of speed, you are going to lose the stability of the skill.

Take walking for example. If you were to jump on a treadmill and walk at 3.5 mph, you would not likely feel fatigued. If you increase your pace, your walking patterns would get more and more out of control with each increase of pace (remember, you are walking at this point, not running). This is the point at which you have lost stability in your skill at walking. If you were to continue increasing your pace, the only thing you could do to keep from being thrown off the treadmill would be to begin running, which is a completely different skill that is separate but related to that of walking.

This is true with any motor skill you can think of. Whether you are writing, shuffling cards, dribbling a ball, paddling a kayak—at some point you are going to cease to have control of your movements if you start trying to do any of these activities at a pace that's too fast for your nervous system to keep up.

Reaction

Reaction is the time between a given stimulus and the beginning of a movement in reaction to that stimulus. In Krav Maga, your reaction time is very important when it comes to how well you respond to an attack or violent situation. Every time you are required to defend yourself you are reacting to an attack that someone else is throwing at you. The sooner that you are able to detect and identify an attack, the more likely it will be that you will defend against it and counterattack in time. The sooner you defend against an attack, the better advantage you will have in fighting back while keeping yourself safe. This is true for an attack that comes upon you by surprise as well as an attack that you were able to detect beforehand.

There are a few kinds of stimuli that you need to be aware of. The most common stimulus that you have to react to is visual, meaning that which you see. When someone throws a punch your way, you see it coming, defend or dodge, and return with a counterattack. Another stimulus that you need to be aware of is auditory, or what you hear. Learning to practice with this sense will allow you to hear someone or something approaching you that does not sound normal or is out of place. Chapter 18 offers more information and training drills.

ESSENTIAL

Training to respond to an audible stimulus can be achieved by reacting to a bell or buzzer during your drills. If you have a partner, you can react to her verbal command. Lastly, try reacting to feeling or touch by having a partner come from behind and try to put you in a headlock, bear hug, or push from behind.

16 CORE TRAINING

Core training has become a common methodology within the fitness world, even though there is a bit of controversy as to what core training really is. Some people think core training is nothing more than abdominal work. However, core training is learning how to move from your midsection. Instead of working just your abs, you are working all of the stabilizer muscles in your shoulders, hips, and spine. Building up your core strengthens the area of your body where nearly all movement begins. And movement is a very important skill to develop as your Krav Maga skills progress.

Concepts of Core Training

The muscular system of your body works in a synergistic fashion. What this means is that it takes more than one muscle to perform a movement. A bunch of muscles working together are required to perform a certain movement. For example, when you perform a bicep curl you must hold some form of weight firmly with your hand while tucking your elbows into the sides of your body. You then bend your arm, squeezing your bicep muscle, which exerts enough force to bring the weight up and lower it back down. To perform even a single bicep curl, far more than just your bicep muscles are working to bend and straighten your elbow while maintaining a seminatural posture. The muscles surrounding the shoulder girdle are required to stabilize your shoulder joint. The muscles in your forearm (and there are a lot of them) work hard to assist the movement of the elbow and maintain the firm grip necessary to keep the weight in your hand.

The next time that you are in the gym doing bicep curls, lateral raises, or any other standing exercise, notice what is happening to the muscles in the trunk of your body. If you make an effort to be observant, you will feel that your core muscles are recruited to stabilize your body, counteracting not only the momentum of your body motion but also the gravitational force of the weight you are moving.

Stabilization

Stabilization is a major component of core training. If you can learn how to get these core muscles to recruit or fire more often with movement and during exercise, you will notice that all of your strength and endurance activities will increase to a higher level of performance. Think of the core of your body as a foundation. Once you have a strong foundation, all of the added parts will have a much better base from which to work.

Core Movement

Although the muscles in your core stabilize your pelvis, shoulder girdle, and spine, they are also required to move these same areas. The core muscles must be strong enough to distribute your body weight, absorb and transfer forces placed upon the body, and generate force to move through your daily activities.

Stabilizing your core muscles also strengthens them—your core stabilizes your body, which allows you to do the exercise. You cannot have one without the other, which goes back to the idea of appropriate progressions. There is a certain amount of stability needed to strengthen, yet there is also a certain amount of strength needed to stabilize. In order to be as mechanically efficient as possible, you have to train for both.

Importance of Core Training

The musculature of your core is an important part of the protective mechanism that relieves your spine from excessive or harmful forces that occur during your daily activities. Individuals who have chronic lower back pain are likely not activating their core muscles on a regular basis. Without activation of these muscles, there is an increased amount of pressure on the disks in your spine as well as an extensive amount of compression force in the lower parts of your spine. Without providing proper core support for your spine, damage can result to the ligaments that support it. Furthermore, this can lead to narrowing of the openings in the vertebrae that the spinal nerves pass through. Nerve compression can be responsible for a condition commonly known as sciatica. When this occurs there is pain, numbness, and tingling all the way down the leg.

Spinal Stenosis

Nerve compression could be the result of spinal stenosis. This disorder often affects one or more of three specific areas in your spine—the canal in the center of the column of bones (the spinal column) where the spinal cord and nerve roots are located, the canals at nerve base or nerve roots where nerves begin to branch away from your spinal cord, or in the spaces between your vertebrae where many nerves go from your spine to other parts of your body. Spinal stenosis can affect a small or large area of your spine.

If it causes pressure on the lower part of your spinal cord or nerve roots, it may give rise to pain or numbness in your legs. If the pressure hits the upper part of your spinal cord near your neck, then it may produce similar symptoms in your shoulders as well as your legs.

Impact Resistance

While training in Krav Maga you will likely receive punches or kicks to the midsection of your body. You need to be able to contract or harden your core muscles so these strikes do not do serious damage upon impact. To make these reactions occur in order to avoid injury takes practice and training.

The core is not solely restricted to your belly region; it extends to the regions of your rib cage and along the back of your body. One of the most common injuries suffered by all kinds of pro fighters is bruised, cracked, or broken ribs. One of the things that protects your ribs and provides them with support is the tight musculature that surrounds them. By strengthening these muscles and training them to harden quickly, you can decrease your chances of suffering fractured ribs that are caused by impact.

Musculature of the Trunk

There are a number of primary muscles that are found within your core. The most common muscles in the core are the abdominal muscles. These are the "six-pack" muscles that are in the front of your body and are the primary core muscles that nearly everyone seeks to develop, often for reasons of appearance. These muscles work to curl your spine forward, as you would do while performing any basic abdominal exercise.

Under the abdominals are your internal and external obliques, which run diagonally across the front of your body. These are the muscles that, when developed, give someone that V-shaped look about the torso. The job of the obliques is to rotate your spine as well as to flex it from side to side (a movement you will commonly perform when dodging, bobbing, slipping, or ducking a punch).

Deep Muscles

There are a number of core muscles many people do not know about. For example, you have the *transversus abdominis* (or transverse abdominal muscle), which runs around the front of your belly much like a belt. This muscle is what allows you to draw your navel inward toward your spine. You are not able to see this muscle as easily as the abdominals simply because this is considered a "deep" muscle in the body. If you have a distended (or swollen) belly, and you are not pregnant, it may be that you have a weakened transverse muscle.

The back of your body has a considerably large and dense muscle—the *quadratus lumborum*, or QL for short. This muscle is part of your lower back and is somewhat like a natural weight belt. This muscle begins at the bottom of the rib cage and comes down to the top of the pelvis. It helps with lateral flexion, rotation, and works to stabilize your spine and pelvis.

> **QUESTION**
>
> **What are deep muscles?**
> Deep muscles are in close proximity to the interior side of your spine, making them almost imperceptible on your body's exterior. The primary deep muscles are *transversus abdominis*, the *multifidus*, and the muscles of your pelvic floor. These deep muscles play a role in stabilization but not in movement.

This muscle is utilized with every punch and kick delivered, so strengthening the QL is a great way to strengthen your punches and kicks. Usually, this muscle is strengthened by general physical exercise, but squats are a great exercise to strengthen your QL. Integrating trunk rotations into quadricep exercises, such as lunges, will also provide an added amount of strength for your core muscles.

More Muscles of the Trunk

Along the bones of your spinal column are layers of muscles that overlap one another. These are called the spinal erectors, and it is very important to keep these muscles physically sound. The closer these muscles are to bone, the smaller they are. As they grow further away from the spine, they begin to increase in length and mass. Whenever you keep the muscles closest to your bones strong, then your joints will have better odds of remaining healthy, strong, and injury free. Exercises that work on extending your spine are excellent for strengthening these muscles—such as the Cobra pose or Bridges. (Refer to the yoga poses section in Chapter 5 for more information.)

As you continue to move down your spine you come to the musculature of your pelvic floor. Your pelvis is shaped like a bowl. The only thing holding the internal parts of your body from falling out of the bottom of this bowl is a layer of muscle known as the pelvic floor. These muscles are highly important, especially in women, for maintaining physical strength. Pelvic muscles are the root of your stability and movement.

You may have already heard of a thing called Kegel exercises, which can help strengthen your pelvic floor muscles. These muscles, like any other, can become weak, and while exercising such weaknesses can become problematic. When performing exercises such as squats or lunges, focus some attention to the tightening of those muscles. This can help you add stability and strength to your entire core and foundation.

QUESTION

What are Kegel exercises and why are they called that?

Kegel exercises are named after Dr. Arnold Kegel. Kegel designed them to strengthen the *pubococcygeus* muscles. The exercises consist of clenching and unclenching the muscles forming part of the pelvic floor (referred to as the Kegel muscles). Factors such as surgery recovery, pregnancy, recently giving birth, and/or weight issues can all result in weakening of pelvic muscles. Kegel exercises help regain pelvic floor muscle strength so that a recently postpartum woman can retrain her pelvic floor muscles to their prepregnancy strength and tone.

Another core section of your lower body is the collection of muscles that cross your hips.

185

Although it may not immediately seem so to you, many of the muscles in your upper legs actually continue to run across your hip joints, helping to stabilize your pelvic region. Due to the role they play in pelvic and hip stabilization, these are considered core muscles as well. Therefore, exercises that strengthen your upper legs, such as leg lifts, cross extensions, lunges, and squats, fall within the scope of core training exercises.

Core Muscles of the Ribs and Shoulders

Moving up your rib cage you will find a tight network of muscles surrounding your ribs. These muscles are referred to as the *serratus* (shortened name), *serratus anterior*, *serratus magnus*, or (because they are active during the action of punching) the "boxer" muscles. The *serratus* run along the side of your body and can be located at a spot that is roughly just below your armpit. The *serratus* muscles are extremely important in the stabilization of your torso. They also work to stabilize and move the housing and components of your shoulder blades, as they connect the front side of your upper body to the back side. Many exercises can engage these muscles, particulary pushups, pull-ups, and chin-ups. You might also try performing sit-ups with your arms over your head, as doing so will engage and therefore help to strengthen your *serratus*.

Lastly, the *latissimus dorsi* (from Latin meaning "the widest of the back"), or "lats" for short, are core muscles. The lats are very large, fan-shaped muscles that are found on either side of the spine on the mid to upper back of your body. Fanning away from the spine, these muscles wrap around the side of your body up to the front and insert at your upper arm bone. The job of these muscles is to perform pulling actions. However, they also play a large part in the stabilization of your spine and shoulder girdle.

Exercises such as rows or pull-ups and chin-ups are excellent for strengthening these muscles. Surprisingly enough, during pushups your lats help to support the entire upper half of your body.

Core Exercises

When training to strengthen your core, you should begin by teaching your trunk how to stabilize itself first before moving onto strength exercises. As with any muscle, too much too soon could lead to injury—and an injury to your core is devastating to any training program. Once you have begun to build power and stability within your core, only then should you begin the core strengthening exercises. Don't forget to focus some of your attention to your pelvic floor; keep it slightly engaged by squeezing the buttocks together.

If you have these muscles properly engaed, you should feel a slight pull inward from your belly button. However, be sure that you do not over do this as internal strains can be quite painful. This pull should be a simple, subtle draw inward of your belly button. This is engaging your lower abdominal wall and *transversus abdominis*.

There are a couple of reasons it is important to strength train the core in this way. First, when holding the pelvic floor and core musculature together you are strengthening your body from the inside out. This is the deepest level of strength training that can be practiced. When this kind of strength is developed you will see an increase in strength in everything you do, from lifting your child into her car seat to your Krav Maga workout routines.

The second reason it's beneficial to train the core this way is that with practice your body will begin to make these muscles fire more frequently whether you are aware of them or not. You want this to become second nature to you, something you automatically do all the time. So when you punch and kick you may not be thinking about how the muscles in the core are firing, but they will be firing due to the fact that you train them. Thus your punches and kicks will naturally become stronger and more powerful.

On the following pages are some exercises for core trunk stability.

Plank

1. Start out on your hands and knees with your hands directly under your shoulders.
2. Step your feet back hip width apart so that you are holding the top of a pushup position.
3. If you are struggling to hold this position, step your feet wider than hip width to distribute the force over a wider base of support.

This exercise is static, which means that you do not move. Your body should be one straight line from your heels all the way up through the top of your head. The entire front body should work to support you. ▼

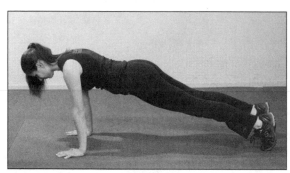

▲ PLANK
Plank is done with both hands and feet pressing into the floor.

SAFETY

Here's a tip to maintain a straight posture in Plank: Pretend there's a string tied at the base of your spine that runs up your back and is being pulled tight at the crown (top of head). This visualization is often helpful to avoid the beginner mistakes, such as drooping your midsection to the ground, lifting your head up, or arching your back. Also keep your navel pulled in slightly.

Yoga Pushup

1. While remaining in the Plank position, lower your body in one straight and solid piece all the way down to the floor. Brush your upper arms and elbows into your ribs as you lower.
2. Once lowered, press with your arms to push yourself back into your starting position (Plank).
3. Return to starting position. The idea is that you do not lose any stability in the trunk of your body as you lower yourself down and return to the starting position. Your arms have to do some of the work here, but try to see if you can make your legs and core take more of the force so that you don't feel as though all of the heavy exertion is being placed on your upper body. If you feel you cannot hold your body, continue practicing Plank and doing pushups on your knees until you feel like you are strong enough to move to pushups on your toes. ▼

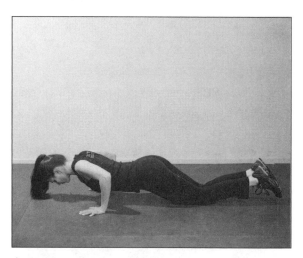

▲ YOGA PUSHUP
You can modify this pose by placing one knee on the floor.

Side Plank

1. Assume a stable and straight Plank position, then step your right hand to a point on the floor that is under your nose.

2. Slowly rotate your entire body all the way to the left (counterclockwise). You must use the inner and outer edges of your feet to stabilize yourself. Your left foot is just in front of your right foot.

3. Next, place your left hand on your hip and take deep, controlled breaths. Once you have achieved balance, be sure that you are using your core by lifting your hips toward the ceiling.

4. Once you can do this with control and balance, try reaching your left arm up toward the sky. Lower the nonsupport (left) arm back down to the floor as you come slowly back into plank position.

5. Now switch sides. If the Side Plank is a little too much for you in the beginning, modify the pose by doing do it with one knee down on the floor. If you are looking to add a little more difficulty, try stacking your feet one on top of the other. ▼

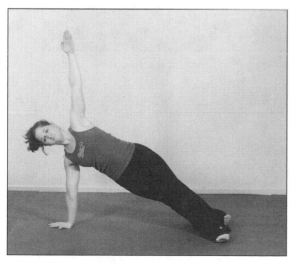

▲ SIDE PLANK
This strengthens the side of the torso, the upper body, and the hips.

Following are some core strength and resistance exercises:

Seated Balance

1. Sit with your feet out in front of you and knees bent.

2. Lift one foot up off the ground followed by the other.

3. Try to lengthen the spine and open up the chest.

4. With both arms parallel to the ground, turn the palms up and reach the arms forward.

5. Try holding for at least 5 seconds in the beginning, then build up to at least 30-second sets. ▼

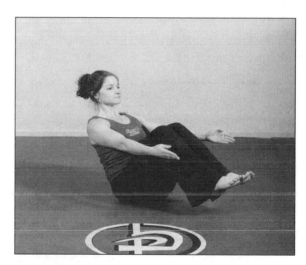

▲ SEATED BALANCE
Great for core strength and stability.

189

Straight-leg Sit-ups

1. Start seated with both legs straight and your arms reaching up toward the ceiling. Inhale.
2. As you exhale, reach your arms forward. Try to round your back down one vertebra at a time, while allowing the arms to move out in front of you.
3. Inhale as you reach your arms over your head.
4. Exhale as you reach your arms forward and peel your body up off the floor to come back to your starting position.
5. You can begin with 4–5 reps, and as you become stronger work up to 10–12 repetitions per set. ▼▶

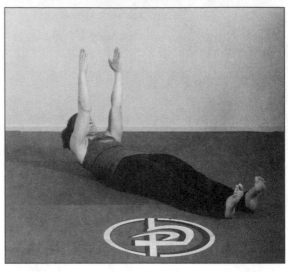

▲ STRAIGHT-LEG SIT-UP #2
Lift with control.

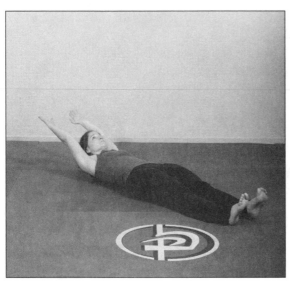

▲ STRAIGHT-LEG SIT-UP #3
Peel your body off the floor without lifting the legs.

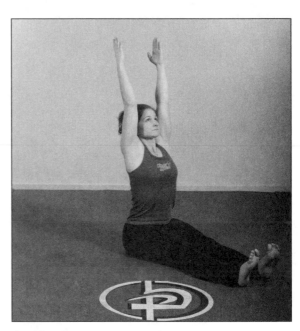

▲ STRAIGHT-LEG SIT-UP #1
Extend the spine and reach up.

Cross Extensions

This exercise is a variation of the classical bicycle exercise.

1. Place your hands behind your head.
2. Without pulling on your neck, take your right elbow to your left knee.
3. Extend your right leg all the way out along the floor.
4. Alternate back and forth while keeping your shoulders from touching down between each repetition.
5. Start with a total of 10 repetitions and work your way up to 20–30. The slower you perform the exercise the fewer reps you will do until reaching a point of muscular fatigue. ▼

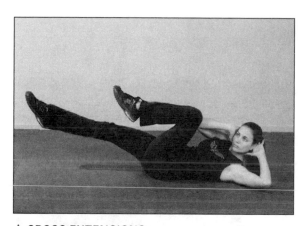

▲ CROSS EXTENSIONS
Great for strengthening the abdominals and obliques.

Half Cross Extensions

1. Lay down on your back, face-up, with your right arm overhead and left leg straight along the floor.
2. As you exhale, touch your right hand to your left toe.
3. Inhale back into your starting position and repeat.
4. Be sure to perform the same amount of repetitions on both sides.
5. Begin with sets of 5–8 reps and build up to 8–12 reps per set. ▼

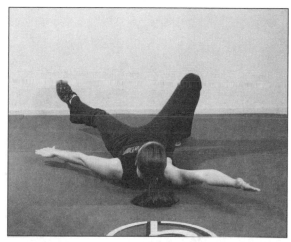

▲ HALF CROSS EXTENSIONS #1
Lengthen the arm and legs away from you.

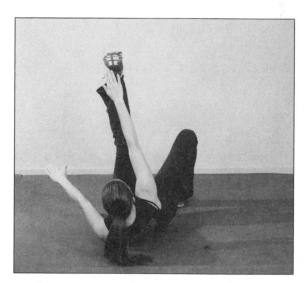

▲ HALF CROSS EXTENSIONS #2
Come up and touch the hand and foot to each other.

Russian Twists

1. From a seated position, balance with your feet lightly touching the floor.
2. Rotate your torso and touch your hands to the floor on one side of you.
3. Reach your hands up and over to the other side.
4. Repeat 8–12 reps per set.

This exercise can also be done with a medicine ball or a hand weight for added resistance. ▼

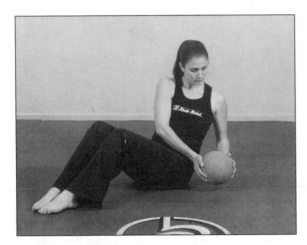

▲ RUSSIAN TWISTS
Strengthens abdominals, obliques, and lower back muscles.

Knee Drive

1. From Plank, lift your right leg up and bring your knee in toward your chest.
2. This can be performed fast or slow, although it's much more challenging when done slowly.
3. Try to keep your shoulders over your wrists when bringing your knee forward.
4. Extend your leg back slowly and place your foot gently on the ground in order to move to the other side.
5. This may be challenging at first. Once you become stronger and more flexible this exercise will become much easier. Start with 6 repetitions per set and build up to 10–12 reps per set. Again, the slower you go the more challenging it becomes to do more repetitions. ▼

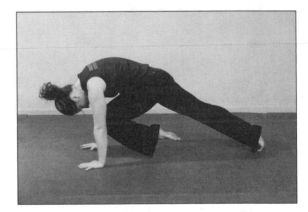

▲ KNEE DRIVE
This exercise can be very intense when done slowly.

Bridge

1. Lay face up, and bend your knees with your feet close to the buttocks and hip width apart. Try to keep your feet parallel to each other (although it may be hard to tell because you should not be able to see your feet).

2. Press the hips up with your legs. You can either hold this as a static exercise or you can lift and lower for repetitions.

3. Ground fighters do a variation of this exercise by rolling over one shoulder and reaching the opposite arm across and back (see the Bridge Variation photo).

4. This exercise should be done at least 8–12 times. You can do a static hold for 5–30 seconds as well. ▼

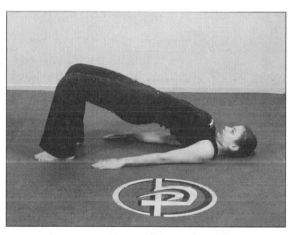

▲ BRIDGE
Strengthens legs and lower back.

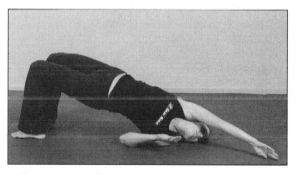

▲ BRIDGE VARIATION
Teaches how to use your hips to get your attacker off of you.

Spinal Extension

1. Lay face down with your elbows in and your hands close to the shoulders.
2. As you inhale, lift your head, chest, and arms off the floor.
3. With an exhale, lower back down toward the floor. Many people look forward when performing this exercise. Keep the chin down so the back of the neck is long.
4. Repeat this 6–10 times. ▼

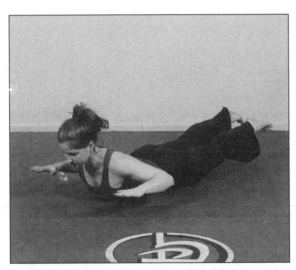

▲ SPINAL EXTENSION
Strengthens the muscles that run along the spine.

For any exercises in which you are training to increase the power in the core of the body, you should perform at least ten to fifteen repetitions and two to three sets of each exercise. Remember when training for power that the exercises are generally done faster than when training for stability or general strength. Keep all of the muscles in the trunk firm when performing any core exercises.

Sit-ups

When performing a sit-up to increase the power of the muscles in the trunk, it is best to anchor your feet either under a sit-up bench or any stable object you can fit your feet under or by using a partner to hold your feet.

There are many variations for the arms. The simplest version is with your arms across your chest. You then sit back so the lower to mid back touches the floor but the shoulders do not. This is different from a regular sit-up in that you are working on power, which means by using your legs to stabilize you can speed up the movement to increase the workload. If that feels easy, try placing your hands behind your head, but be sure as you come up you do not pull your head forward to assist your sit-up. Lastly, you may hold a weighted ball at your chest or overhead to increase the resistance. Remember, whenever you add speed it should be just enough to also stay in control of the exercise in both directions, in this case sitting up as well as going back. ■

194

Double Leg Lifts

1. Lying on your back, find something to anchor your hands down with. You may grab your partner's ankles or the legs of a chair. Just be sure whatever you use is heavy enough that you do not lift it off the ground.

2. Take both legs up toward the ceiling, keeping your legs as straight as you can. Make sure your naval is moving toward your spine. If your hamstrings are tight, you may have to bend your knees to bring your legs to this position.

3. Inhale as you lower your legs down as far as you can without the spine moving from its starting position.

4. Your legs will come back up at the last half of your exhale.

Once you have found your range of motion you can begin to speed up the pace of the exercise. You may lose the stability of the spine slightly. This is probably fine for someone who has a healthy back and spine. However, if it bothers your back, slow down and only work through the range of motion that does not irritate your back or feel painful. Once you have built up some strength in the midsection you will find that your range of motion will increase. ▶

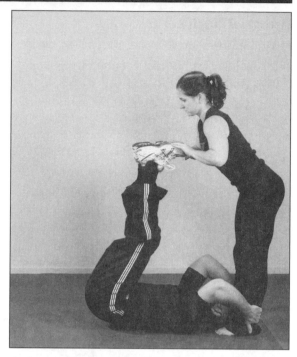

▲ DOUBLE LEG LIFTS #1
Start with the legs up.

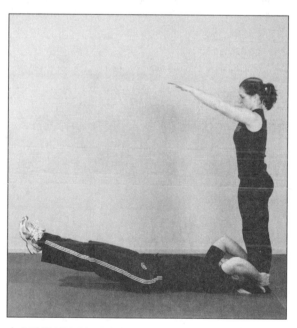

▲ DOUBLE LEG LIFTS #2
Lower the legs and bring them back to the starting position.

195

CHAPTER 16   CORE TRAINING

Overhead Rotations

This is a great exercise to strengthen all of the muscles in the mid section of the body.

1. Stand with a medicine ball at your left thigh.
2. Reach the ball out to the left side, up over your head, and down to the right side.
3. Finish with the ball touching the right thigh and repeat in the opposite direction. ▼▶

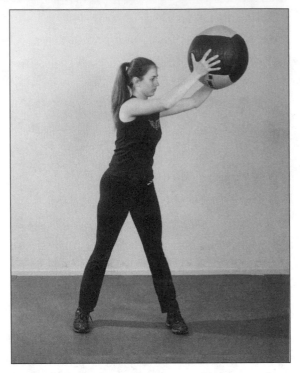

▲ OVERHEAD ROTATIONS #2
Reach the ball out then up

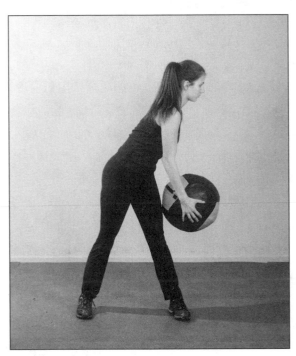

▲ OVERHEAD ROTATIONS #1
Start with ball at thigh

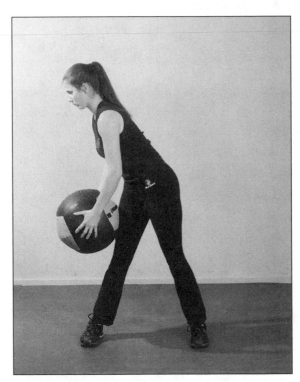

▲ OVERHEAD ROTATIONS #3
Finish with ball at thigh

196

Crunch-ups/V-ups

This is an old gymnastics exercise. Once you are able to perform a Seated Balance, you are ready to try Crunch-ups.

1. From the Seated Balance position, inhale as you extend your legs out and exhale as you bring them back.

2. Start with your hands on the floor, just next to or behind your hips, then try holding your arms parallel to the floor.

3. Once you've mastered this, try the exercise with straight legs. The upper and lower body will both lower toward to floor without touching, you then come back up and reach toward the toes. This is called a V.

4. Drop back and burst up, staying balanced and finding a rhythm that works for you. ▼▶

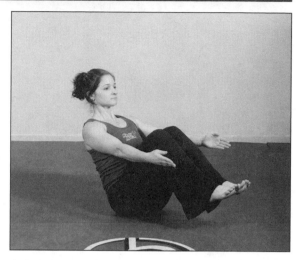

▲ CRUNCH-UPS #2
Come up by bringing your knees toward your chest.

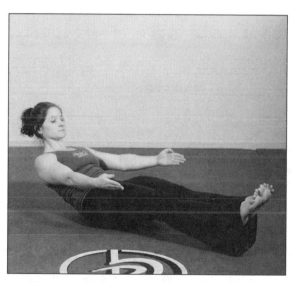

▲ CRUNCH-UPS #1
Start with arms and legs extended.

197

17 STARTING YOUR KRAV MAGA WORKOUTS

If you are new to Krav Maga (or to any exercise), it is important to allow your body to adapt slowly to the demands placed on it. It is recommended you start with the beginner formats at least two to four times per week for the first two weeks before moving on to intermediate formats. You may experience some muscle soreness after your first couple of workouts. This amount of soreness should subside if you remain consistent with your training sessions. With practice, the movements will begin to feel more natural and easier for you to perform.

When learning Krav Maga techniques, it is important to remember that you want to learn the movements before going all out with your punches and kicks. Newer students have the tendency to try too hard and often end up battling with their own bodies' mechanics in an attempt to make strong attacks (which may cause you to become injured). Stay relaxed, breathe, and try not to overthink your movements. Once you have learned the proper training and technique, the power of your attacks will come naturally and will not have to be forced. This will reduce your risk of muscle soreness and injuries from overstressing your body.

The following formats include many components of physical fitness in addition to beginner Krav Maga movements. If you do not understand any part of the workout instructions, the chapter where the exercise was introduced is cross-referenced so you can find a detailed description on how to execute the exercise, movements, or drills.

The Warm-up

Alternate walking for 1 minute with jogging for 1 minute around the block, park, or room for a total of 10 minutes. If you are not able to jog, make it a brisk walk. The goal is to get the body temperature and heart rate to increase slightly. It doesn't matter what activity you choose; any cardiorespiratory activity will do.

The following sequence focuses on lower body strength, balance, and coordination as well as opening up the hips. Take your time as you work through the following two-three sets of exercises:

- 10 Basic Squats with arms forward (Chapter 6, page 66)
- 10 reps total alternating High Knee Holds (Chapter 8, page 100)
- 10 reps total alternating Straight Leg Lifts (Chapter 8, page 101)
- Stationary Lunges, five reps on each leg (Chapter 6, page 71)
- 10 pushups with knees down ■

Warming Up Your Core

This segment helps to open and strengthen the hips a bit more. It also helps to strengthen the muscles in the legs and core of the body. Move in and out of these stretches to help the muscles release a little at a time while increasing blood flow to the areas being lengthened. You may feel it challenging to stay balanced while rotating. This is a good thing. Take your time and focus as you rotate the torso.

Torso Warm-up Routine:

1. Plank for 10 seconds (if you cannot hold it for 10 seconds, hold it for 5, come down, and do it again). (Chapter 16, page 188)
2. Step your right foot through your hands to a Runner's Lunge Low. With hands on hips, lift torso upright and hold this stretch for the front of the hips for 5–10 seconds while taking deep breaths. (Chapter 5, page 51)
3. Hold the Low Lunge and rotate your torso to the right. Hold the rotation for 5–10 seconds and breathe.
4. Hamstring Stretch. Move your upper body down toward the front leg while keeping your spine long and your sit bones moving behind you. Hold for 10 seconds. (Chapter 5, page 53)
5. Externally Rotated Runner's Lunge. (Chapter 5, page 52)
6. Step to Plank, hold for 5–10 seconds.
7. Repeat with your other foot forward. ■

Core Strength Segment

The following segment is great for increasing core strength and increasing strength and mobility in the spine. Try to follow the recommended breathing pattern. The breathing will initiate the next movement. You may hold a position for more than 1 breath.

1. Start in Plank and control your breath. (Chapter 16, page 188)
2. Exhale as you lower body to the floor, keeping your elbows in to your ribs.
3. Inhale as you move into Cobra, hold for 3 cycles of breath (Chapter 5, page 53)
4. Exhale as you move into Downward Facing Dog, hold for 5 breaths. (Chapter 5, page 50)
5. Inhale and return to Plank.
6. Repeat 4 times.
7. After the last Downward Dog, walk your hands back to your feet.
8. Hang in Forward Fold for 3 cycles of breath. Bend your knees slightly if needed. (Chapter 5, page 54)
9. Roll up slowly. ■

Functional Training Segment

This will begin the cardio and combative portion of your workout. Try to keep moving. If you feel like you are working too hard, slow down and focus on taking deeper breaths. Remember, you want to try to keep your heart rate up at a moderate intensity. Try to fall into a rhythm when working on your punches as this may help you to count out your combinations.

Remember to keep your hands up, recoil your punches, and to rotate your torso while punching. Make sure that you are using the muscles in your legs in order to drive your punches into the target.

Punch Combo 1

Before beginning this workout, review Chapter 13 for the fundamentals of punching. From a regular Fighting Stance:

1. Left Straight Punch 10 times (Left Jab)
2. Right Straight Punch 10 times (Right Cross).
3. Left-right combo 10 times.
4. Left-right-left-right combo 10 times.
5. Left-right-left-right-left-right combo 10 times.
6. Nonstop alternating Straight Punches for 20 seconds.
7. Left-left-right combo.
8. Left-left-right-left-right combo.
9. Nonstop Straight Punches for 20 seconds (you can mix it up).
10. Repeat in the opposite Fighting Stance. ■

Kick and Knee Combo 1

Again, find a rhythm. If you feel like you want to do more than ten that's fine. Sometimes it takes a few practice knees before your body finds the correct timing. Repeat this entire sequence two times total:

1. Right Knee Strike 10 times.
2. Left Knee Strike 10 times.
3. Right Front Kick 10 times.
4. Left Front Kick 10 times.
5. Right Round Kick 10 times.
6. Left Round Kick 10 times. ■

Ground Combo 1

In this segment, be sure you set a solid foundation before beginning your kicks. These are great exercises for training balance and coordination on the ground and strengthening the muscles in the core. Repeat this sequence two times:

1. Right Side Kick from the Ground 10 times. (Chapter 14, page 170)
2. Left Side Kick from the Ground 10 times. (Chapter 14, page 170)
3. Bridge ten times. (Chapter 16, page 193)
4. Cross Extensions 20 times. (Chapter 16, page 191)
5. Roll to Seated Balance 5 times. (Chapter 16, page 189)
6. Russian Twist 10 times. (Chapter 16, page 192) ■

Stretch Segment

This stretch segment will lengthen the muscles in your hips and lower back. Hold each stretch for about thirty seconds and focus on making your exhale breaths long and relaxed. Final stretch and cool down:

1. Lay face-up with your knees to your chest.
2. Release your right foot to the floor.
3. Reach your left foot to the sky for the left Hamstring Stretch. (Chapter 5, page 53)
4. Do a Thread the Needle stretch to the left. (Chapter 5, page 56)
5. Bring your left knee to your chest with your right leg straight on the floor.
6. Do a Spinal Twist, left knee drops to right as head looks left. (Chapter 5, page 56)
7. Bring both knees to your chest.
8. Move to the other side. ■

Stretch Segment Part 2
1. Begin in Child's Pose. (Chapter 5, page 50)
2. Lying face down, grab the top of one foot, just as in the Standing Quad Stretch. (Chapter 8, page 101)
3. Switch sides and repeat stretch on opposite leg.
4. Return to Child's Pose.
5. Move into a Downward Facing Dog. (Chapter 5, page 50)
6. Walk your hands to your feet.
7. Hang in Forward Fold, remember to bend your knees if necessary. (Chapter 5, page 54)
8. Roll up slowly. ■

After Your First Workout

Congratulations on finishing your first Krav Maga fitness workout! Keep in mind that you may experience some muscle soreness over the next couple of days. If you feel like you are too sore to exercise, this means you may have overdone it. Perhaps you should take the time to recover before your next session. If you only feel slightly sore, do only some sort of cardio training the following day to loosen up the tight sore muscles.

This workout is slightly more challenging than Krav Maga Fitness Format A. It is recommended you do Format A at least three times before moving into Format B. Some of the skills in Format B are slightly more complex and take more coordination. Take your time with learning the movements, then begin to pick up the intensity of the workout.

The Warm-up

Warm up with any of the following, repeating for six minutes:

- 30-second brisk walk
- 30-second jog
- 30-second skip with high knees
- 1-minute fast walk, 3-minute jog ■

Remember that the goal of this portion is to increase body temp and heart rate. If you feel as though you cannot complete the full three minutes of jogging, then walk when needed. Make reaching the allotted time your goal.

Warming-up for Format B

The following exercises will open the hips, train dynamic balance, and strengthen the lower body. Remember to keep your spine lifted and elongated. Perform two to three sets of the following exercises:

1. Standing Quad Stretch, 10 times each leg. (Chapter 8, page 101)
2. Alternating Runner's Lunge stepping back 10 times. (Chapter 5, page 51)
3. Spinal Twists 10 times total. (Chapter 5, page 56)
4. Lateral Lunges 10 times. (Chapter 6, page 72)
5. Sumo Squats 10 times.(Chapter 6, page 66)
6. To finish, hold the Sumo Squat and press your thighs out with elbows for five seconds. ■

Building Upper Body Strength

These exercises will increase the strength in the upper body and shoulder girdle. They also build strength in your spine as well as the muscles in the trunk of your body. Repeat two to three times:

1. Downward Dog for 5 breaths. (Chapter 5, page 50)
2. Hands to floor, step back to hands and knees.
3. 5 pushups, making sure your elbows are tucked in.
4. 5 pushups with hands wide (place your palms slightly more than shoulder width apart).
5. Lower to floor until torso comes to rest.
6. Reach your arms up and forward while raising your legs off the floor into the Spinal Extension position. Hold for roughly 2 seconds.
7. Roll over onto your back.
8. Cross Extensions 20 times. (Chapter 16, page 191)
9. Bring your knees to your chest, roll up to Seated Balance (back and forth) 5 times. (Chapter 16, page 189) ■

Lengthening and Strengthening Segment

This sequence is great for opening and lengthening all of the muscles in the backside of the body. It also teaches the body how to stabilize the core and builds strength in the upper body. Remember to use the breathing pattern. Repeat the following sequence five times:

1. Downward Facing Dog for 5 breaths. (Chapter 5, page 50)
2. Inhale to Plank. (Chapter 16, page 188)
3. Exhale as you lower body two inches from the floor, keeping your elbows in to your ribs.
4. Inhale as you push back up to Plank.
5. Exhale to Downward Facing Dog.
6. Repeat 4 times.
7. After the last Downward Facing Dog, walk your hands back to your feet.
8. Hang in Forward Fold for three cycles of breath. Bend your knees slightly if needed. (Chapter 5, page 54)
9. Roll up slowly. ∎

Working the Whole Body

This next segment incorporates lots of variables. It opens the hips and lower back, back of the legs, and shoulders. It strengthens the upper body, the lower body, and trains static balance.

1. Step right leg forward into a Runner's Lunge, reach arms overhead and hold 2–5 seconds while breathing deeply. (Chapter 5, page 51)
2. Lower right knee to floor into Runner's Lunge Low. (Chapter 5, page 51)
3. Open and reach both arms out to sides, opening the chest and the front of the body.
4. Release and come across with the right arm pulling in toward your chest with the left arm. Hold for five seconds.
5. Bring hands to floor, extend right leg into Hamstring Stretch. (Chapter 5, page 53)
6. Reach left arm to outside of right knee 5 times.
7. Return to Runner's Lunge, with arms up. Hold for 5 seconds. (Chapter 5, page 51)
8. Bring hands to mat, step into Downward Facing Dog (Chapter 5, page 50).
9. Repeat on the other side with left arm and leg. ∎

Moving Your Feet

Do not rush through the following segment. The footwork is important here, and you want to be sure that you are using your lower body to move in the desired directions. Be sure to stabilize your landing before going to the next movement.

1. Begin in Fighting Stance. (Chapter 13, page 146)
2. Advance and retreat 10 times.
3. Move right and left 10 times.
4. Repeat in opposite Fighting Stance ■

For detailed instructions on the following techniques, please refer back to Chapters 13 and 14.

1. Begin in Fighting Stance. (Chapter 13, page 146)
2. Left Straight Punch 10 times. (Chapter 13, page 149)
3. Right Straight Punch 10 times.
4. Left Straight Punch with advance, traveling forward 10 times.
5. Left-right Straight Punches with advance, traveling forward 10 times.
6. Repeat in opposite Fighting Stance. ■

SAFETY

Remember: The punch opens as the lead leg moves. The punch closes or recoils as the second leg returns to a fighting stance. This takes practice to learn the correct timing.

Training For Lower Body Attacks

Ideally, you want to do this while traveling across an open area. Perform two to three sets of the following:

- Alternating Knee Strikes, traveling forward 10 times. (Chapter 14, page 165)
- Alternating Front Kicks, traveling forward 10 times. (Chapter 14, page 160) ■

Wrapping Up

Take your time with this sequence. You may find it challenging to stay balanced at first. Keep practicing. Your balance will improve, as will your dynamic flexibility. Be sure you are pivoting your base foot on the round kicks. This sequence will get the heart rate up! Repeat the following sequence two to three times:

1. Squat into alternating Front Kicks 10 times. (Chapter 14, page 160)
2. 3 stationary Front Kicks left leg (3 steps to other side) then right leg, 8 times total.
3. Left Front Kick, two left Round Kicks, (3 steps to other side), then right leg 8 times total. (Chapter 14, pages 160, 162)
4. 10 Left Side Kicks (move into kick with a step). (Chapter 14, page 166)
5. 10 Right Side Kicks. ■

Working the Core

For the following exercises, try moving from one exercise to the next without resting. It is put together in a way that you should not need to stop. Repeat the following sequence two to three times:

1. Seated Balance 10 seconds (try to extend your legs). (Chapter 16, page 189)
2. Half Cross Extensions 10 times each side. (Chapter 16, page 191)
3. 3 Side Kicks on the Ground, then flip to other side, 8 times total. (Chapter 14, page 170)
4. Bridge 10 times. (Chapter 16, page 193)
5. Straight-leg full Sit-ups 10 times. (Chapter 16, page 190) ∎

Cool Down

Take some slow, deep breaths and enjoy the time you are cooling down and relaxing. These exercises will open the hips, spine, and lower back. For more detailed instructions on how to perform cool-down exercises properly, please refer back to Chapter 8.

1. Sit cross-legged.
2. Fold forward.
3. Switch cross of legs.
4. Fold forward.
5. Seated single-leg Forward Fold. (Chapter 5, page 54)
6. Twist to the other side.
7. Seated single-leg Forward Fold.
8. Switch legs.
9. Happy Baby (Chapter 5, page 55). ∎

Remember to always be aware of your breathing and never hold your breath while exercising (this can cause you to develop a hernia, among other things). To review breathing techniques, please refer to Chapter 5.

18

KRAV MAGA TRAINING DRILLS

You should think of your Krav Maga fitness in broader terms than simply the static physical attributes that you acquire. Measure your Krav Maga fitness by the degree at which you have mastered the drills. Drills are the method you use to learn how to control your body. In keeping with Krav Maga's idea of fitness, you must train your mind as well as your body, and you must train them to work together. Properly designed drills will train you to perform efficiently and effectively while under high levels of stress and fatigue. Feel free to mix and match the pieces: learn to combine techniques, integrate exercises, and switch your training emphases in different ways.

Technique Drills

Technique drills are simply those drills designed to improve your ability to execute proper technique and form. They can be done either standing or while on the ground. Keep in mind that technique drills pertain to the physical mechanics of how you perform a punch or a kick. Training at a slower pace is a great way to practice Krav Maga movement during the beginning period of your training. This enables you to recognize when and where you may be losing a part of the technique. Slowing down allows you to feel your own mistakes, which you can then correct throughout your performance. Movement drills can be as simple or as complicated as you would like or need them to be for your level of training.

Repetition is another way to enhance your Krav Maga movements. Repeating a technique creates a motor pattern in you body that makes it easier to perform that action again. When you practice something over and over again with improper technique, you are accentuating improper technique. It's key to practice repetition of movements with proper alignment in order to avoid injures and to move efficiently and effectively every time you do the technique. Remember, a solid foundation will support a bigger building. Your fundamentals are your foundation. Practice them well and practice them regularly.

The Alternating Straight Punch Drill

1. Stand in a Neutral Stance with your feet a little wider than shoulder width apart. (Chapter 13, page 146)
2. Even though you are not in your regular Fighting Stance, you will still begin by throwing (at a slow pace) alternating Straight Punches. (Chapter 13, page 149)
3. Concentrate first on rotating your shoulder girdle while keeping your elbows down and in toward your ribs. Breath at a continuous and even pace.
4. Once you feel you are able to do that without much conscious thought, concentrate on using your legs and lower body to rotate your pelvis and shift your hips forward with each punch. The more ability you have to use your feet to generate force from the ground up, the stronger and more solid the delivery of your punch will be.
5. Feel your weight shift from one leg to the other.
6. Make sure you make adjustments as needed during moments when you feel unstable or off balance.
7. Continue to check that the position and posture of your body are correct. Reminder: The punches move out and back. The shoulders and hips are rotating. The legs are being utilized and are transferring weight forward into each punch. Stay loose and relaxed. With practice it should begin to feel effortless. ∎

8. Once you've got this routine down, change from Straight Punches to Hook Punches, then proceed to Upppercut Punches. (Chapter 13, pages 149–155)

9. Do either 2–10 punches of each type, or repeat different punches for about 30 seconds at a time. (Remember, this is a drill to practice technique. How many repetitions you perform is not the goal.)

Adding Difficulty

An advanced version of this alternating punch drill is to throw two alternating (switching from one hand to the other) Straight Punches followed by two alternating Hook Punches and finishing the combo with two alternating Uppercut Punches. Continue this cycle without pausing for a total of thirty seconds, then progress to sixty seconds and so on. To increase the intensity of this drill, at the end of each cycle, add an exercise such as dropping into a pushup position and completing a set of 5-10 pushups, then get up quickly and repeat the cycle of punches again.

Build up your level of speed only as long as you can maintain quality in your techniques and posture. Slow training is very valuable in preparing your body to work, especially when you use it as a warm-up. Training slowly is also excellent for mastering proper balance and footwork. Mistakes are hard to spot when you are executing at full speed. Whenever you slow your movements down, however, all your weaknesses and bad habits will be made far more apparent, allowing you a chance to rectify them.

SAFETY

When increasing speed, be careful not to lose control of your techniques. Speed must be coupled with control in order to be effective. An out-of-control technique will be less effective, no matter how fast it is executed.

The Advancing Straight Punch Drill

This drill is used to pratice the timing of moving forward and punching simultaneously. As you push off the back foot the front foot moves you forward. When the front foot lands on the floor the punch should be extended all the way out. Recoil the hand and bring the back foot into a Fighting Stance to finish. Continue this exercise moving forward in repetition. ▼ ▶

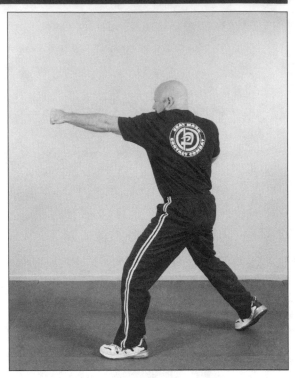

▲ ADVANCING STRAIGHT PUNCH #2

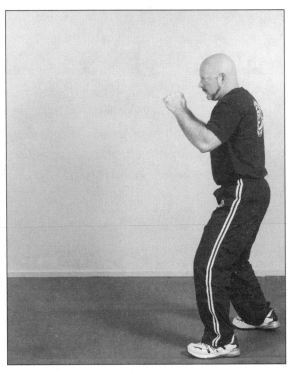

▲ ADVANCING STRAIGHT PUNCH #3
This drill combines a straight punch combination and a forward advance with your feet.

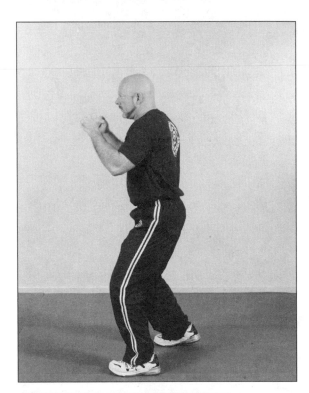

▲ ADVANCING STRAIGHT PUNCH #1

212

The Advancing Left-Right Combo Drill

This drill combines a left-right combination of Straight Punches and advancing forward with the body into one attack. The idea is that you are able to burst in and close the distance between you and your opponent while delivering punches at the same time.

1. Find an open space where you can walk about 10 paces.
2. Begin in your Fighting Stance with your left foot forward and go through the following steps as you say to yourself what you are doing along the way. (Chapter 13, page 146)
3. As your left hand begins to travel forward to deliver the punch, the left foot moves forward. At the same time the right leg and foot will push off the ground to move the entire body forward in space.
4. Your punch will be fully extended (as if you are making contact at that point) while the front foot lands on the ground. The left punch and the left foot land simultaneously.
5. As you begin to recoil your first punch, your rear foot presses into the ground to rotate your back hip forward as you send your rear-hand Straight Punch.
6. As your second punch recoils, check your stance, weight, and balance before doing it again. Both feet should be on the ground when any punch is extended all the way out.
7. Be sure your hips are driving your weight forward and your shoulder girdle rotates with each punch. ■

Once you are comfortable with the pattern and the timing of this movement, try keeping your feet as close to the ground as possible. You should glide along the floor rather than jump into your punches. You can then begin to burst forward and explode into you punches.

As a beginner, you should practice this drill a few times every day, if possible, for at least a few minutes at a time and with enough intensity to muster a sweat. Start with just an advancing jab, then follow up this combination with other combatives as you become more comfortable with it.

Even though you see words such as "explode" and "burst," it is important for you to remember to stay in total control of your body movements by keeping yourself at a low-speed pace. Imagine the speed and try to create the sensation of power with your mental intensity. The whole point of slow training is for you to build a strong foundation of Krav Maga fundamentals (a balanced stance, effective use of movement, and clean striking techniques). This foundation requires balance, motor skills, and effortless, automatic execution.

Hooks and Uppercuts

This drill is used to develop the movements involved in mechanically correct Hook and Uppercut punches. Hooks and Uppercuts are more complex movements due to the fact that one joint (the elbow) remains fixed while the other joint (the shoulder) moves freely. These two punches are almost the same punch, they just move through different planes. A Hook Punch is delivered on the transverse plane whereas the Uppercut is delivered on the vertical plane.

Using a partner helps you alter the angle between punches and makes this drill more dynamic. But you can certainly get a similar effect by using a rope that is hung from your ceiling, dangling a balloon or tennis ball on a string, or sticking a pole or stick into the ground in front of you (make sure it stands at shoulder level).

When using a partner, you should begin at a distance of just over an arm's length for safety. As you become more comfortable and advanced, you may close the distance. The distance may also need to be altered depending on what techniques are being practiced. For example, if a drill involves elbows, then it will not do to be at an arm's distance.

214

Hooks and Uppercuts Drill

1. Begin facing each other in a Fighting Stance about one arm's distance away from each other. You may adjust your distance when you get going. Your partner will hold his arm either parallel to the wall or parallel to the floor, depending on the punch being executed, with a 90 degree bend in the elbow. Slowly move your hand around your partner's forearm keeping the bend of your elbow at a right angle. At the end of your punch, your bicep should be against your partners forearm.

2. Recoil your punch in the same path you sent the punch. Once you've got the right path, you can pick up the speed.

3. Work up to the point where you send your punch faster, timing your contact and recoil as your bicep barely slaps against your partner's forearm.

Practice this about 10-20 times. This exercise should help you understand the mechanics of the Hook Punch or Uppercut Punch. This is a drill that improves on technique so take your time learning the motion. ▼►

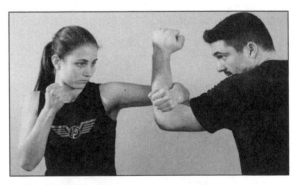

▲ HOOK DRILL
Move your hand around your partner's forearm, keeping the bend of your elbow at a right angle.

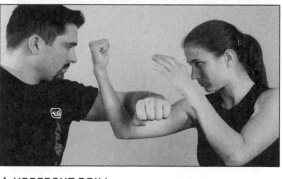

▲ UPPERCUT DRILL
Time your contact and recoil so that your bicep barely slaps against your partner's forearm.

Constant Self-Regulation

Make any necessary adjustments before you continue or repeat this drill. This constant self regulation should always be in your thoughts when you are training with slow work. Remember, when you become your own toughest critic, it will make you more effective at training alone.

After recoil is complete, take a moment to check your stance and ask yourself the following questions:

- Are you ready to make another movement in any direction from here?
- Are your hands up, chin down, elbows in, and eyes forward?
- Is your weight properly distributed?

Reaction Drills

Vision, speed, and reaction drills have a high degree of overlap, as do many things in Krav Maga. Reaction drills include exercises that require you to perform certain tasks based on outside stimulus or cues from a trainer or training partner. These drills will sharpen your ability to react without hesitation, whether it's a ball thrown toward you, a car pulling in front of you, or a violent situation in which you need to defend yourself.

ESSENTIAL

The use of loud audible cues is good for reaction drills. There are a wide range of possibilities when it comes to the cues you use. Try having your partner slam something down or smack a pair of focus mitts together, anything that causes a sudden loud sound. Audible cues are excellent since they help you to pinpoint targets more quickly by using your hearing.

Reaction drills work somewhat on the principle of give and take. For example, you throw a punch and your partner blocks it, or your partner presents a focus mitt and you strike it immediately. The cues of your reaction drills can be visual (seeing a punch being delivered.), audible (a word, whisper, scream, or sound), or tactile (being pushed or grabbed).

215

What You'll Need:

■ Partner

■ Punching/kicking shield

Start out in Neutral Stance. Your partner stands directly in front of you with the kick shield held tight to his or her chest. Wait for your partner to move the kick shield in front of you at the same time they yell a cue, such as "go!" When you see the shield and hear the cue, deliver a proper front kick to the pad.

Building on the Reaction Drill

To build from here, your partner will randomly move the bag slightly to either side of him instead of just in your direct front. Your goal is now to kick the shield with your same-side leg that the bag moves to (this will add a component of recognition to your drill).

ESSENTIAL

Reaction drills can be done with an almost unlimited number of combinations of combatives and cues. Some combinations might make more sense than others, so find combinations that you can relate to your own reality or that you feel flow well together.

To add even further difficulty to this drill, your partner can also move the shield into positions for Round Kicks or pick up the pace.

For more advanced training, have your partner move around with the bag. This will force you to add movement to your combatives. Another added difficulty is to have your partner begin calling out numbers from one to nine (or to as high a number as you desire). Your goal is to throw the number of kicks that your partner calls in rapid-fire succession.

If you do not have a kick shield there are other ways to do the same type of drill. With focus mitts your partner can slap them together and call even numbers two through ten. When you hear the number and see the mitts, you send that many Straight Punches (see Chapter 13) to the mitts. If you only have a heavy bag, your partner can call out the numbers while you react to her cue and send that many punches to the bag. Be creative with the equipment you have. The same drill will work while shadowboxing.

Fatigue Drills

As the name suggests, these drills are designed to train your mind, as much as your body, to perform past the point of exhaustion. The focus is more about continuing past the point when you think you can't continue than proper form.

When faced with an attack on the street in which you have to fight for your life, within seconds hormones are released in your body that can be exhilarating but also totally exhausting. You cannot stop fighting in a real life situation because you are tired. These drills train you to continue the fight until you are safe no matter how fatigued you may be.

Fatigue Drill 1

You will need a partner and a punch shield.

1. Throw nonstop Straight Punches to the shield. (Chapter 13, page 149)
2. When your partner cues you, drop and do 5 pushups.
3. Burst back up onto your feet and throw nonstop punches again.
4. Continue this drill for a total of 60 seconds. Once you have built up some endurance, increase the time in increments of 30 seconds. ■

Fatigue Drill 2

For this drill you will need a medicine ball of proper weight as well as enough space for you to move about freely enough to perform the drill without obstruction.

1. Perform pushups with the medicine ball until your partner yells "go!"
2. Sprint down to where your partner is standing with a kick shield and perform ten strong Front Kicks. (Chapter 14, page 160)
3. Sprint back to your medicine ball and repeat pushups until your partner calls the next cue.
4. Continue this drill for a total of 2 minutes.
5. Increase the difficulty by alternating from kicks to punches each time you return to the punch/kick shield. ■

You can increase the number of kicks or punches you throw at the shield, and you can increase the time you perform the drill. To make it interesting, try vertical jumps, pushups, squats, or tossing the medicine ball between the kicks and punches. Mix it up!

Fatigue Drills

217

CHAPTER 18 KRAV MAGA TRAINING DRILLS

Stress Drills

While fatigue can certainly be considered stress, it is not necessarily the only factor that causes stress in a fighting situation. Krav Maga uses the term *stress* to refer to elements of a fight, such as getting pushed or hit, avoiding obstacles, being injured, or simply being in unfamiliar surroundings.

Your body responds when it is hit or punched, especially when it hurts. This can make it very difficult for you to make decisions and react instantly. Stress drills are exercises that should make you uncomfortable (not only from fatigue, but from unexpectedness) and demand instant reaction and repetition.

React to the Unexpected: The Sudden Stress Drill

For this drill you will need a partner and a punching/kicking shield.

1. Stand passively with your eyes closed (no peeking!).
2. Your partner stands in front of you and shoves you with the bag, then holds it for a front kick counterattack.
3. When you feel the bag hit you, open your eyes and attack with a Front Kick or a rapid-fire series of Front Kicks. (Chapter 14, page 160) ■

This drill is great for training vision, recognition, and reaction. It does not have to be restricted to Front Kicks alone. As you become more comfortable with the drill, incorporate other combative such as knees and punches

Adding Intensity

Here are some ways you might increase the level of stress:

■ Turn down the lights.
■ Allow your partner to approach from behind and from different, more unorthodox, angles.
■ Increase the power behind you partner's attack and your counterattack. ■

Standing with your eyes closed when you know an attack could come at any moment can be a bit unnerving, but training will help you greatly overcome your fear. The idea is to breathe deep and to think nice, calming thoughts while waiting for your partner's shove. Doing so will increase the level of surprise when you get shoved, simulating the reality of being attacked while off guard.

As always, remember that you are training. The power behind the shoves you receive from your partner should increase slowly as you proceed through the drill. Eventually, you want those shoves to have enough force behind them to knock you off balance. They should not be rough enough to cause injury to you or your partner.

ESSENTIAL

Physical methods that will help you learn to exhibit mental intensity or aggression include furling your brow, growling, and gritting or baring your teeth. These expressions are throwbacks from our predatory past and may help you find an inner aggressiveness or power that you never knew you possessed. This is inner power is what martial artists refer to as your fighting spirit.

Never be deliver these shoves to someone's head or other sensitive areas. After all, your eyes are closed and, consequently, your risk is mildly increased. Start light and verbally ask for small increments of additional power behind the shoves, but only when you are ready for them. Remember to talk to your partner—he or she is not the enemy. If your partner increases the power of the shoves a little too much, do not hesitate to tell him or her to bring it back down a notch.

Stress Drill 2

Equipment needed: focus mitts.

1. Stand in a Fighting Stance with your forearms covering your head. (Chapter 13, page 146)
2. Your partner is going to make you uncomfortable and use the mitts to disturb you by poking or lightly hitting you with the mitts in your midsection, your ribs, and maybe toward you head and arms.
3. Your job is to absorb the attacks and keep your eyes open.
4. When you partner slaps the mitts together, he will call out even numbers (two through ten), and you send that many punches to the mitts and go right back to absorbing the hits. ■

This drill will keep you from cowering in a fight. It teaches you to be aggressive under a stressful situation and to keep your eyes open so you can see what is going on. Make sure your partner starts lightly with only a few attacks at a time. As this becomes less stressful for you, your partner can pick up the amount of attacks or increase the amount of force within each attack.

What Is Mental Intensity?

This means exhibiting an intense state of mind while maintaining precise mental acuity. If you are in a threatening or violent situation on the street where you have to defend yourself, it is vital that you allow your fighting spirit out by being aggressive. You may not have experienced this emotion before. During training, try to release that aggressive side no matter how uncomfortable it may feel (especially if it's new to you). This way if it is ever needed, you can rest assured that you know it's there for you to tap into.

ALERT

Those who are not familiar with fighting tend to react to sudden aggression by freezing up. This reaction is comparable to a deer freezing in headlights. Stress drills are excellent for fighting against this tendency. When done with even a minor level of regularity, these drills will effectively minimize your odds of having a deer-in-the-headlights reaction when attacked without warning.

All of these Krav Maga drills are designed to improve your chance of survival in a difficult situation. These drills increase your confidence in techniques by giving you a chance to succeed under stress, they help decrease reaction time, and they increase your strength, endurance, and ability to function under stress in the context of a fight. While performing these drills it is necessary to emphasize aggressiveness. Even if you think you did something wrong or are not sure of a technique, perform it with conviction and confidence. Once predators see a sign of weakness in you, they will take advantage of the situation. Training at being aggressive will translate to situations on the street.

Why Train Under Stress?

When or if you ever find yourself in a situation in which you are being threatened or attacked, your body experiences a certain type of stress or pressure. When the mind and body are placed under this stress, it becomes hard to make quick decisions and reactions to keep yourself safe. Krav Maga training drills try to simulate what it would be like to find yourself in an actual life-threatening situation and teach you to react appropriately, which is why it's important to add some kind of stress to your training drills.

19 INTERMEDIATE KRAV MAGA WORKOUTS

At this point you might find yourself making certain mistakes in your Krav Maga technique. Don't be discouraged by this. The fact that you are beginning to recognize your mistakes means that you will be able to correct them. You should also find that you are better able to recognize when, where, and how you are making these mistakes. The upside to this awareness is that you will be able to self-regulate your Krav Maga sessions and make corrections when you need to.

The Warm-up

Start with a one-minute fast walk or a two to three minute jog. Repeat this two to three times depending how you feel. If you feel you need to warm up a little more, then definitely do it a third time. Sometimes at this point in training it feels good to run a little more. If you find that this is the case, go for it. Pay attention to and follow what your body is telling you to do.

The following sequence is going to get your heart rate up in small bursts. Remember to take deep breaths when your heart rate begins to increase. Take as little time as possible from one exercise to the next. Most of these exercises emphasize agility, so remember to focus on switching directions quickly.

Warm-up

Repeat sequence two times:

1. Double-Leg Lateral Hops 15-20 seconds. (Find a line, or place something down on the floor such as a rope or belt. Keeping your feet together jump back and forth over the line. Work on being light on your feet and increasing the speed.)
2. Single-Leg Lateral Hops on each leg 15–20 seconds. (Same action as above but on one foot.)

3. Lateral Touch 10 times total. (Place two cones on the floor about three feet apart from each other. Touch the first cone and move laterally to the other cone. Continue back and forth changing directions as quickly as possible working on agility.) ■

Functional Training Segment

Try to move quickly into the next sequence, the functional training segment of the workout. The upper and lower body will work at the same time. Remember to keep the muscles of the core region engaged. That means pulling in the navel slightly, engaging the pelvic floor, and holding the abdominal wall firm.

This sequence requires a medicine ball. It is recommended for women to start with a four-pound ball then move up to a six-pound ball within a couple of weeks. Men should begin with a six- to eight-pound ball. If you do not have a weighted ball, you can use a basketball or any other ball, even a hand weight will work.

Training Sequence 1

Equipment needed: medicine ball or weight
Repeat this sequence 2–3 times:

1. Squat with overhead reach 10 times. (Chapter 6, page 66)
2. Alternating Runner's Lunge, stepping back holding ball in front of chest 10 times total. (Chapter 5, page 51)

3. Overhead Rotations 10 times total. (Chapter 16, page 196)
4. Wood Choppers, 5 times each side. (Chapter 7, page 88)
5. Lateral Lunge (hold ball under one arm) 5 times each side. (Chapter 6, page 72) ■

The following sequence begins to warm up the shoulders and the upper body with pushups, generates some power in the legs with jumps, and opens up the hips with some dynamic, active stretching. Take your time with the exercises that require you to stand on one leg; they can be challenging. Stay focused and control your breathing.

Training Sequence 2

1. Pushups, hands wide, 10 times.
2. Knee Drive 10 times total. (Chapter 16, page 192)
3. Vertical Jump 10 times. (Chapter 6, page 69)
4. High Knee Hold 8 times total. (Chapter 8, page 100)
5. Standing Quad Stretch with floor touch 8 times total. (Chapter 8, Page 102)
6. High Knee Hold 10 times total.
7. Sumo Squats, slow with hands at sternum, 8 times. (Chapter 6, page 66)
8. Static Sumo Squat for 10 seconds. (Chapter 6, page 68)
9. Hands to floor, walk hands forward to Downward Facing Dog. (Chapter 5, page 50)
10. Repeat. ■

Stretch Segment

This is a sequence that emphasizes movement with breathing. Notice the breathing pattern and try to be consistent with it as you go.

Stretch Segment

1. Downward Facing Dog. (Chapter 5, page 50)
2. Inhale to Plank. (Chapter 16, page 188)
3. Exhale and Lower to floor.
4. Inhale to Cobra. (Chapter 5, page 53)
5. Exhale to Downward Facing Dog.
6. Step right foot through to High Runner's Lunge. (Chapter 5, page 51)
7. Arms overhead (inhale), hands to sternum (exhale), right rotations 3 times.
8. Hands down on mat, step to Plank (inhale), lower to floor (exhale).
9. Cobra (inhale) to Downward Dog (exhale).
10. Step other foot through hands and repeat other side.
11. After the last Downward Dog, walk your hands back to your feet.
12. Hang in Forward Fold for 3 cycles of breath. Bend your knees slightly if needed. (Chapter 5, page 54)
13. Roll up slowly. ■

Intermediate Krav Maga Combatives

Spinal rotations begin the foundation of the movement you will continue using in Krav Maga punches. Use the same rotation of the shoulder girdle and pelvis to send your punches as you do in your spinal rotations.

Intermediate Comabtives

1. Spinal Twists 10 times. (Chapter 5, page 56)
2. Alternating Straight Punches 10 times. (Chapter 13, page 149)
3. Alternating Hook Punches 10 times. (Chapter 13, page 153)
4. Alternating Uppercut Punches 10 times (Chapter 13, page 155)
5. Repeat 2–3 times. ■

You can work these combinations to the heavy bag or focus mitts, in which case you would need a partner to hold for you. Have you or your partner go through the entire sequence then switch pad holders. If you do not have mitts or someone to hold for you, you can shadowbox the combination.

Punch Combo Drill (to focus mitts)

Punches are straight punches unless otherwise specified.

1. Left-right combo.
2. Left-right-left-right combo.
3. 10 Left Hooks. (Chapter 13, page 153)
4. 10 Right Hooks.
5. Left-right-left Hooks.
6. 10 Left Uppercuts. (Chapter 13, page 155)
7. 10 Right Uppercuts.
8. Left-right-left Hook, right Uppercut.
9. Left-right combo, then bob and weave to right side (pad holder swings left arm).
10. Left-right combo, bob and weave, right Cross.
11. Left-right combo, bob and weave, right Cross, left Hook.
12. Left-right combo, bob and weave, right Cross, left Hook, right Uppercut. ■

Intermediate Combatives for the Lower Body

Now to work the lower half of your body. As you perform the following techniques in repetition, try to find and maintain a rhythm that is comfortable for you. You can do these either to a pad or just move through the motions. The technique is slightly different with each. When you are not making contact to a pad you have to keep from driving your weight into the attack to stay in control.

Lower Body Combatives

1. 10 Right Knee Strikes. (Chapter 14, page 165)
2. 10 Left knee strikes.
3. 10 Right Front Kicks. (Chapter 14, page 160)
4. 10 Left Front Kicks.
5. 10 Right Round Kicks (Chapter 14, page 162)
6. 10 Left Round Kicks. ■

Training to Fight

This drill is done to simulate a round in a fight. If you are working with a partner and using mitts, the person holding the mitts will call out numbers one through four and the puncher sends that many alternating straight punches with as much power as possible. Work like this for one minute. Increase the time of the round as your training progresses. This drill should feel very challenging on your cardio system. Once you are comfortable with straight punches you can add in other variations. The idea is that the puncher has to react to what the holder cues. If you are not working with a partner, cycle through the punches for the length of time desired. You may also add in:

- Double Jab
- Strong Right Cross
- Right Cross, recoil, Right Cross
- Single Hooks and Uppercuts

Intermediate Core Training

You can't forget your core! Move from one exercise to the next with little to no rest. Perform two to three sets of the following sequence:

Intermediate Core Training

1 10–12 Straight leg Sit-ups.
2. 10–12 Sit-ups.
3. 10–12 Russian Twists. (Chapter 16, page 192)
4. 10–12 face-up Leg Lifts. (Chapter 8, page 101)
5. 10–12 Crunch-ups. (Chapter 16, page 197)
6. Cross Extensions 20 times. (Chapter 16, page 191)
7. 10–12 Spinal Extensions. (Chapter 16, page 194) ■

Final Stretch

Take your time with the final stretch. Enjoy lengthening your muscles and breathing. See if you can make your exhales longer than your inhales to relax deeply.

Final Strech

For your final stretch:

1. Lay face down and grab your right foot (Standing Quad Stretch). (Chapter 8, page 101)
2. Switch sides.
3. Push back to Child's Pose, step right foot forward into Low Lunge. (Chapter 5, pages 50, 51)
4. Shift hips back to right Hamstring Stretch. (Chapter 5, page 53)
5. Move forward to Low Runner's Lunge. (Chapter 5, page 51)
6. Lift left knee off floor.
7. Inhale to Plank. (Chapter 16, page 188)
8. Exhale to floor.
9. Inhale up for Cobra. (Chapter 5, page 53)
10. Exhale to Child's Pose, hold for 5 breaths.
11. Repeat sequence with left leg.
12. Stand up with feet wide.
13. Perfrom Knuckles Behind Back, hinge forward at hips. (Chapter 5, page 57)
14. Step feet together, do Eagle Arms on both sides. (Chapter 5, page 57) ■

225

The Warm-up

Now you can mix up the beginning of your warm-up with jogging, running, jump rope, and shadowboxing. If you are still not sure how to shadowbox, do some of the combinations from the past workouts. There is no need to move fast. Take your time and work on shifting your weight, moving your head, and using your legs.

Warm-up

1. Light jog for 2 minutes.
2. Fast jog for 3 minutes.
3. Run or jump rope for 3–5 minutes.
4. Slow dynamic shadowbox for 2 minutes. ■

The arm swings in the following sequences are shown with a kettle bell in Chapter 7. The same swing can be performed with two- to ten-pound hand weights. The idea is to generate power and muscular strength at the same time holding the core muscles together to help stabilize the spine.

Using a heavy weight:

1. 10 Double-arm Swings
2. 10 Basic Squats with rotation, alternating right than left. (Chapter 6, page 66)
3. 5 Lateral Lunges to right then left. (Chapter 6, page 72)
4. 5 Single-arm Swings right then left.
5. 10 Alternating Lunges stepping back with arms overhead.
6. Shadowbox for 2 minutes. (Chapter 14, page 171)
7. Repeat sequence 2–3 times. ■

Stretch Segment B

The first stretch in this sequence combines two positions. The wide stance forward fold with the knuckles behind the back is to open the shoulders. There is one Downward Facing Dog in this sequence that is held for a long period of time. When performing any yoga posture for a long period of time, be sure you are breathing with full inhalations and exhalations. As you inhale in Downward Facing Dog, try to lengthen the pose. As you exhale, try to deepen the pose as you press your hips back with your legs firm. Sink into your heels. If this is not restful, bend your knees.

Active/Static Stretch

1. Stand with your feet wide, Knuckles Behind Back (Chapter 5, page 57), hinge forward at hips.
2. Flat back (hands on shins).
3. Roll up to stand.
4. Wide leg Forward Fold (Chapter 5, page 54), hands to floor.
5. Reach the torso toward the right leg, hold for 5 seconds, then toward the left leg and hold 5 seconds. Then bring the hands back to the center.
6. Walk hands and feet into Downward Facing Dog, hold for 60 seconds. (Chapter 5, page 50)
7. Walk hands forward into Plank position (inhale) (Chapter 16, page 188)
8. Move to Side Plank (Chapter 16, page 189) and hold for 3 breaths. Repeat each side 2 times.
9. Move to Plank (exhale).
10. Lower to Cobra (inhale). (Chapter 5, page 53)

11. Move to Downward Facing Dog (exhale). (Chapter 5, page 50)

12. Step right foot between hands and straighten the spine, then reach to the sky with your arms and balance.

13. Bring left hand to floor next to arch of right foot, reach right arm to sky (twisting right) and hold for 5 seconds. Release the right hand down to the floor.

14. Step to Plank (inhale) and exhale into position.

15. Inhale to Cobra.

16. Move to Downward Facing Dog (exhale).

17. Repeat each side 2 times.

18. From Downward Facing Dog, walk hands to feet/legs to Forward Fold.

19. Place hands down on mat and step feet back to Plank.

20. Do 5 Yoga Pushups, walk hands back to feet to Forward Fold. (Chapter 16, page 188)

21. Finish last set in Forward Fold position, hold for 5 breaths.

22. Return to standing position. ∎

Hold each one of the following positions for two seconds then release:

- Dynamic stretch (Chapter 5, page 49)
- 10 alternating High Knee Holds. (Chapter 8, page 100)
- 10 alternating External Rotation Holds. (Chapter 8, page 100)
- 10 alternating Leg Lifts. (Chapter 8, page 101) ∎

Basic Krav Maga Fight Combinations

Combinations are the heart of Krav Maga fitness training. The basic 1–4 fighting combinations are done on a heavy bag. Practice rotating the body, shifting the weight from left to right while delivering a powerful attack every time you make contact. You will have to learn this movement slowly at first, but once the movement pattern has been learned you can make your attacks fast and strong.

The numbers in the combinations represent how many alternating straight punches you deliver, starting with the left hand and ending with the opposite leg round kick from your last punch. The combinations are as follows:

1. Basic 1: left punch, right kick
2. Basic 2: left-right punch, left kick
3. Basic 3: left-right-left punch, right kick
4. Basic 4: left-right-left-right punch, left kick

The basic 2 and 4 combinations are more technically challenging than the 1 and 3. The reason is that you are required to send the left kick, which is the forward leg, and it has less travel time to gain momentum. Your left kick is usually not going to feel as strong as your right leg kick unless you work on making them both strong through training and practice.

Heavy Bag Combos

1. Start in Fighting Stance. (Chapter 13, page 146)
2. 2, 4, and 6 alternating Straight Punches for 60 seconds. (Chapter 13, page 149)
3. Right leg Round Kicks. (Chapter 14, page 162)
4. Switch stance.
5. 2, 4, and 6 Straight Punches for 60 seconds.
6. Left leg Round Kicks, 10–15 repetitions ■

1. Start in Fighting Stance. (Chapter 13, page 146)
2. Basic 3, 10 reps.
3. Basic 1, 10 reps.
4. Combine basic 3 and 1, 10 reps.
5. Flip to the other side. ■

1. Start in Fighting Stance. (Chapter 13, page 146)
2. Basic 2, 10 reps.
3. Basic 4, 10 reps.
4. Flip to the other side. ■

Repeat the following drills two times:

Bursting Drill

1. 10 seconds slow work.
2. 10 seconds fast work for a total of 60 seconds. ■

Drilling with Combinations

First begin with the following prep:

Repeat twice on each side:

1. 10 Right Knee Strikes. (Chapter 14, page 165)
2. 10 Left Knee Strikes. (Chapter 14, page 165) ■

Combination Drill

You can do as many rounds of the following as you feel appropriate for your fitness level. Begin with at least two and move up from there. You should take about one minute to recover between each round. As you become more physically fit, you will notice your need for recovery time will decrease. This is a great drill for fighters as well as cardiorespiratory training. Perform two-minute rounds of the following:

1. In order, basic 1, 2, 3, 4.
2. 3 Right Knee Strikes. (Chapter 14, page 165)
3. 3 Left Knee Strikes. (Chapter 14, page 165)
4. Repeat. ■

Kicking Drill

This next drill is a way to improve the technique of your kicks. Training kicks in repetition allows you to self-regulate and correct any technique leakages that may occur. Your heart rate will reach your higher zones with this drill. This drill can be performed with Front Kicks and/or Round Kicks.

1. 1 right, 1 left.
2. 2 right, 2 left.
3. 3 right, 3 left.
4. 4 right, 4 left.
5. Repeat second set with the left leg leading. ■

Core Training Format B 1

1. Plank. (Chapter 16, page 188)
2. Right knee to chest
3. Right knee to right triceps.
4. 6 reps total.
5. Switch to the other side. ■

Core Training Format B 2

1. 10 Spinal Extensions with arms reaching forward. (Chapter 16, page 194)
2. 10 seconds in Side Plank. (Chapter 16, page 189)
3. Repeat pose on other side.
4. 5–6 Straight-leg Sit-ups, holding a weight in one hand. (Chapter 16, page 190)
5. 5–6 Straight-leg Sit-ups holding weight in other hand.
6. 10–12 full Sit-ups with weight reaching overhead.
7. Repeat sequence 2–3 times. ■

Final Stretch Format B

Seated with wide legs

1. Reach right, then left, then center.
2. Seated Forward Fold (seated variation). (Chapter 5, page 54)
3. Spinal Twist. (Chapter 5, page 56)
4. Happy Baby. (Chapter 5, page 55)
5. Deck Squat. (Chapter 6, page 70)
6. Roll up to a standing position. ■

Once you are able to get through Format B of the experienced workouts you can then mix and match your workouts. You can take the warm-up, stretches, and combinations that you like and develop your own workout formats. Look back through the chapters and incorporate additional training drills, strength-training exercises, and flexibility techniques that work well for you. Have fun and enjoy your training process!

229

20 NOW WHAT?

Having made it this far, you should now know the basics of what to do, how to do it, and why you should be doing it. All that is left is for you to actually do it. No matter how far you are from your goals, everyone takes the same first step: Begin your first workout and finish it. Before you know it, you'll have accomplished what might have seemed overwhelming to you before you began to work out.

Will It Work For You?

The Krav Maga fitness program is perfect for anyone who wants to get in great shape, inside and out, because it allows everyone to give all they can in each workout. Krav Maga was designed to get anyone into shape, regardless of how fit you are when you start. While it is easy to imagine a beginner hitting a wall of exhaustion after twenty or thirty minutes, even an advanced student can wear himself out in less than thirty minutes. If your goal is to get in shape, follow the guidelines in this book. They have worked for thousands of students, military and law enforcement personnel, professional fighters, as well as older and out-of-shape people. The only difference is the starting point and the desired end result.

The style and design of these training programs are self-regulating. That means that it is up to you to give everything you have for each workout.

Krav Maga fitness training achieves results in your cardiovascular system, builds lean muscle, improves mental focus, relieves stress, and develops real self-defense and fighting skills that may one day save your life. This fun and exciting training system doesn't require any previous fighting experience or fitness level before you get started.

While a young and athletic trainee might throw 2,000 or more combatives in a workout with an average 60 pounds of force, a newer or injured trainee might throw 500 combatives with an average of 20 pounds of force.

Yet both might feel equally challenged and fatigued. What is important is that both pushed themselves to fatigue, triggering their body to improve.

What Are You Waiting For?

Get started right away, and vow to continue for a full thirty days. After that you won't want to stop. Krav Maga training is addictive. While you may struggle through the first few weeks, it will become a healthy habit after just one month. For many, Krav Maga training is the favorite part of their day. Krav Maga classes have become the focal point for many students who take classes four or five days a week, often two to three classes each evening.

The hardest part is getting started, so get started while all this new information is fresh in your mind and your enthusiasm is high. Do something. Procrastination leads to feelings of frustration and disappointment. Starting will immediately improve your mental state.

Benefits of Training at a Krav Maga Training Center

There are several benefits to training at a Krav Maga fitness center. The first and most important is that you will have the vast knowledge of a trained and certified Krav Maga instructor at your disposal.

These instructors are required to go through at least 120 hours of training to achieve Instructor status, and continuing education is required annually.

Another benefit of training at a center is being able to work in a group setting where you can gain experience and understanding from other Krav Maga students. You also get immediate feedback on your techniques while training at a center. So if you are doing a movement improperly, you will be able to rectify your technique before you open yourself up to injuries.

Professional Instructors

Unlike many martial arts and self defense programs, Krav Maga has a rigorous training program that not only evaluates and trains individuals in technique and movements, but also teaches them the principles and teaching methodology that makes Krav Maga so wonderfully effective and easy to learn.

While anyone can open a karate or tae kwon do studio—regardless of rank, qualifications, knowledge, or teaching ability—Krav Maga is a self-defense and fighting system that is internationally regulated to provide a consistently high-quality product. The Krav Maga instructor certification places a great emphasis on teaching ability. Being an excellent practitioner Krav Maga is only half the battle. Being able to transfer the knowledge quickly and effectively is equally important.

Feedback

Getting feedback on your technique is very useful, especially in the beginning. If you have errors in your technique, and practice thousands of times, you build muscle memory and habits that become difficult to change later on. If possible, consider private lessons if the classes don't interest you or are not available given your location or schedule.

Class Camaraderie

Krav Maga classes are exciting and difficult, and they leave you with a sense of accomplishment after each one. (You should feel the same sense of accomplishment after your own workouts.) Many people get additional enjoyment sharing this with their workout partners and the entire class. There is a sort of bonding that takes place. If you feel, as many do, that the group training environment is for you, check out *www.kravmaga.com* for locations throughout the world.

No Excuses

Don't become dependent on a gym environment for training. Mix up your locations as well as the type, duration, and focus of your workouts. You are the product. So depend solely on yourself, and never let yourself down. Avoid the usual excuses: bad weather, long workdays, too much to do.

Learn to train anywhere—outdoors, in cold weather, in hot weather, in the rain. Varying environmental factors will only help to further strengthen you.

Don't Miss a Beat

Trying to fit your training into your busy workday schedule is a recipe for trouble. Consistency is the key to long-term results. Try to train early in the morning, before your day gets away from you and before you get tired or too busy. If you have a predictable schedule that allows for regular training during the evening, then follow that. Having a class that starts and ends at a given time will give structure to your training. If it is truly important, you will find time for yourself.

How to Keep Up Training if You're a Frequent Traveler

Although it may not be the workout you are used to doing, there are plenty of things you can do anywhere and anytime with no equipment: shadowboxing, plyometrics, stretching or yoga, slow work on technique. You can still cross train or do intervals in your hotel room!

Fitting Workouts into a Busy Schedule

If you miss your planned workout, make it up by doing something just before bedtime. You don't need to do anything too serious or strenuous, but if you let yourself go to bed without doing anything, you set a bad precedent that can spiral out of control.

You should make a commitment to working out. You can simply stretch out or pick something you've been neglecting and dedicate a few minutes to that. This way you go to bed feeling a sense of accomplishment and pleased that you didn't let yourself down.

What Brings People to Krav Maga

Krav Maga fitness training really is an all-encompassing and very diverse training program. You will see yoga techniques and postures, movements that look like or are similar to Olympic-style lifting, and different type of modalities that increase flexibility and increase power. Many of these drills professional fighters and athletes use in their everyday training sessions to increase their level of performance.

Greater Skill

Krav Maga fitness training is a great way to increase your skills in Krav Maga, but because of the many training techniques incorporated into this type of exercise program you will notice an increase in performance in every other activity or sport you do as well. In the beginning stages of training you may not understand how many systems within the body are being stimulated from such a well-rounded training system, but with time and practice you will become more aware of how the body responds and is affected by the training drills provided.

Greater Self-Esteem

One of the first things people report experiencing with Krav Maga training is that their self-esteem is drastically increased. There are many reasons for this. First, it's very empowering to punch and kick. It's a skill that many people do not get to do very often if at all. After just one training session you will feel like you are stronger and more able to keep yourself safe should the need arise.

With continuous practice that feeling is maintained, and Krav Maga students begin to walk with better posture and with more confidence than ever before. Research shows that a mugger or aggressor chooses a victim with intent. The person who looks like the victim is the one who is usually the target of an assault. When it comes to self-defense, confidence and self-esteem go a long way.

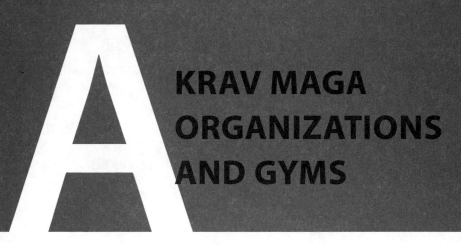

APPENDIX

KRAV MAGA ORGANIZATIONS AND GYMS

ARIZONA

Krav Maga Training Center of Chandler
7200 W. Chandler Blvd. Suite 9
Chandler, AZ 85226
(480) 705-5728

Krav Maga & Fitness
5870 W. Thunderbird Rd. Suite A-3
Glendale, AZ 85308
(602) 866-5728

Krav Maga & Fitness Center of Phoenix
3202 East Greenway Rd. #1635
Phoenix, AZ 85032
(602) 485-5728

The Ultima Martial Arts
6781 N. Thornydale, Suite 219
Tucson, AZ 85741
(520) 744-4591

Ultima Self Defense and Fitness LLC
7649 E Speedway Blvd.
Tucson, AZ 85715
(520) 721-2348

ARKANSAS

Krav Maga & Fitness of Arkansas
10301 Rodney Parham Ste. B4
Little Rock, AR 72227
(501) 779-1737

237

CALIFORNIA

Berkeley Krav Maga Training Center
1500 Ashby Ave.
Berkeley, CA 94703
(510) 486-8000

Kovar Martial Arts, Inc.
7538 Fair Oaks Blvd.
Carmichael, CA 95608
(916) 480-0456

Ceres Karate
2005 Central Ave.
Ceres, CA 95307
(209) 537-5790

America's Best Chatsworth Karate
21360 Devonshire St.
Chatsworth, CA 91311
(818) 772-2467

Universal Martial Arts Center
4200 Chino Hills Parkway, Suite 825
Chino Hills, CA 91709
(909) 597-1710

Modern Combat & Survival Training Center
514 South Corona Mall
Corona, CA 92879
(951) 616-8142

Krav Maga Training Center
7166 Regional Blvd.
Dublin, CA 94568
(925) 829-8430

International Institute of Martial Arts
456 E. Mission Rd.
San Marcos, CA 92069
(760) 591-0456

Core Self Defense
855 Jamacha Rd.
El Cajon, CA 92019
(619) 442-6731

Church's Martial Arts
165 S. El Camino Real, Suite G
Encinitas, CA 92024
(760) 634-3638

Krav Maga Training Center
4040 Papazian Way
Fremont, CA 94538
(510) 490-8300

Valley Fight Club
700 East 7th St.
Hanford, CA 93230
(559) 584-7333

Huntington Beach Krav Maga & Fitness
16889 Beach Blvd.
Huntington Beach, CA 92647
(714) 375-4567

Krav Maga of Orange County
5 Federation Way
Irvine, CA 92692
(714) 876-6256

KM San Diego
P.O. Box 13453
La Jolla, CA 92039
(619) 682-7090

Krav Maga of Orange County
26212 Dimension Way
Lake Forest, CA 92692
(714) 876-6256

Krav Maga of Livermore
1342 North Vasco Rd.
Livermore, CA 94550
(925) 443-3400

Universal Martial Arts Centers
41625 Electric Way, F-1
Palm Desert, CA 92260
(760) 568-0649

California Karate Academy
4000 Middlefield Rd
Palo Alto, CA 94303
(650) 321-2821

Krav Maga of Pleasanton
243-A Main Street
Pleasanton, CA 94566
(925) 846-1700

Krav Maga Rancho Cucamonga
7890 Haven Ave. #6
Rancho Cucamonga, CA 91730
(909) 483-4210

Brand X Martial Arts
432 Maple St., Suites 1 & 2
Ramona, CA 92065
(760) 788-8091

Fight Academy of Rohnert Park
5675 Redwood Dr.
Rohnert Park, CA 94928
(707) 584-3812

MMA Academy
11777 Sorrento Valley Rd.
San Diego, CA 92121
(858) 755-7665

Krav Maga Official Training Center
1455 Bush Street
San Francisco, CA 94109
(415) 921-0612

Krav Maga of San Ramon
2432 San Ramon Valley Blvd.
San Ramon, CA 94583
(925) 837-3040

Get Safe
1288 S. Lyon St.
Santa Ana, CA 92705
(714) 834-0050

Academy of Self Defense
3475 Woodward Ave.
Santa Clara, CA 95054
(408) 844-8485

360 Self Defense
1136 E. Willow St.
Signal Hill, CA 90755
(562) 424-4666

American Martial Arts Academy
6295 Pacific Ave.
Stockton, CA 95207
(209) 952-4000

Xtreme Fit
32820 Wolf Store Rd.
Temecula, CA 92592
(951) 303-8000

One World Martial Arts
33415 Western Ave.
Union City, CA 94587
(510) 663-9675

Shin's Family Martial Arts Center
27674 N. Newhall Ranch Rd. #10
Valencia, CA 91355
(661) 713-9174

Krav Maga of Walnut Creek
1839 B Ygnacio Valley Rd.
Walnut Creek, CA 94596
(925) 932-9000

COLORADO
Boulder Krav Maga
2750 Glenwood Drive
Boulder, CO 80304
(303) 449-2010

Northern Colorado Krav Maga
6821 West 120th Avenue, Unit C
Broomfield, CO 80020
(720) 214-1691

Krav Maga, LLC
3218 Wedgewood Court
Fort Collins, CO 80525
(970) 225-6655

Rocky Mountain Krav Maga
119A Wilcox St.
Castle Rock, CO 80104
(303) 681-2622

Champions Kempo Karate, Inc.
5612 N. Union Blvd.
Colorado Springs, CO 80918
(719) 593-2232

CONNECTICUT

Premier Martial Arts
15 Cheryl Dr.
Canton, CT 06019
(860) 693-9294

Defensive Edge, LLC
13 Summit St. Suite 311
East Hampton, CT 06424
(860) 267-4448

Defensive Arts & Fitness
628 New Haven Rd.
Naugatuk, CT 06770
(203) 723-1907

Connecticut Krav Maga at Breakthru Family Fitness
48 Union Street
Stamford, CT 06906
(203) 355-9395

FLORIDA

Cape Coral
211 Hancock Bridge Pkwy
Cape Coral, FL 33990
(239) 574-5437

Master Clark's Black Belt Academy
9114 Wiles Rd.
Coral Springs, FL 33067
(954) 757-2821

Master Clark's Black Belt Academy
1153 N. Federal Hwy.
Ft. Lauderdale, FL 33304-1423
(954) 567-5686

Master Clark's Black Belt Academy
1019 NW 76th Blvd.
Gainesville, FL 32606-6753
(352) 332-8065

Master Clark's Black Belt Academy
4860 NW 39th Ave.
Gainesville, FL 32606-7235
(352) 337-1396

Master Clark's Black Belt Academy
1400 Millcoe Rd.
Jacksonville, FL 32225
(904) 724-2100

Master Clark's Black Belt Academy
7235 Atlantic Blvd.
Jacksonville, FL 32211-8708
(904) 724-2100

Master Clark's Black Belt Academy
2771 Monument Rd.
Jacksonville, FL 32225-5549
(904) 996-8111

Master Clark's Black Belt Academy
9825 San Jose Blvd.
Jacksonville, FL 32257-5494
(904) 268-4424

Master Clark's Black Belt Academy
14286-10 Beach Blvd.
Jacksonville, FL 32250-1561
(904) 821-0901

Master Clark's Black Belt Academy
13170 Atlantic Blvd.
Jacksonville, FL 32225-6149
(904) 221-3036

Master Clark's Black Belt Academy
9802 Baymeadows Rd.
Jacksonville, FL 32256-7917
(904) 620-9884

Master Clark's Black Belt Academy
4792 Windsor Commons Ct.
Jacksonville, FL 32256
(904) 223-7079

Master Clark's Black Belt Academy
445 State Road 13
Julington Creek, FL 32259
(904) 230-2791

Harmony Martial Arts Center Inc
1928 Commerce Lane, #8
Jupiter, FL 33458
(561) 745-0230

Victory Martial Arts
3855 Lake Emma Rd.
Lake Mary, FL 32746
(407) 444-5636

Victory Martial Arts
3188 Lake Washington Rd.
Melbourne, FL 32934
(321) 752-5600

Master Clark's Black Belt Academy
6800 NW 169 St.
Miami, FL 33015
(305) 558-7252

Darren Buckner's ATA Black Belt Academy, Inc.
529 41st Street
Miami Beach, FL 33140
(305) 672-1350

Master Clark's Black Belt Academy
556 Atlantic Blvd.
Neptune Beach, FL 32266-4024
(904) 241-0100

Master Clark's Black Belt Academy
950-26 Blanding Blvd.
Orange Park, FL 32065
(904) 276-2344

Master Clark's Black Belt Academy
1580 Wells Rd.
Orange Park, FL 32073-2336
(904) 264-7555

Master Clark's Black Belt Academy
1545 County Rd. 220
Orange Park, FL 32003-7922
(904) 264-9111

Victory Martial Arts
150 Alafaya Wood Blvd., Suite #104
Oviedo, FL 32765
(407) 977-5200

Victory Martial Arts
783 North Alafaya Trail
Orlando, FL 32828
(407) 736-0222

Victory Martial Arts
312 E. Michigan St.
Orlando, FL 32806
(407) 648-1690

Victory Martial Arts
13938 Egret Tower Dr. Ste. A
Orlando, FL 32837
(407) 857-0520

Victory Martial Arts
150 Alafaya Woods Blvd.
Oviedo, FL 32765
(407) 977-5200

Master Clark's Black Belt Academy
801 S. University Dr.
Plantation, FL 33324-3336
(954) 424-2337

Master Clark's Black Belt Academy
288-A Solana Rd.
Ponte Vedra Beach, FL 32082
(904) 285-4031

Shuman's ATA Black Belt Academy
18350 Paulson Dr
Port Charlotte, FL 33954
(941) 255-5425

Master Clark's Black Belt Academy
1770 A1A South, Suite D
St. Augustine, FL 32080-5520
(904) 471-3829

Del Castillo Premier Martial Arts
10014 Cross Creek Blvd.
Tampa, FL 33647
(813) 973-4634

Victory Martial Arts
2175 Aloma Ave.
Winter Park, FL 32792
(407) 671-7300

Master Clark's Black Belt Academy
1360 Weston Rd.
Weston, FL 33326
(954) 888-9188

GEORGIA
KBX Gym
1007 Union Center Dr., Suite A
Alpharetta, GA 30004
(770) 777-0845

Canton Krav Maga & Fitness
320 Adam Jenkins Memorial Drive, #100
Canton, GA 30115
(404) 784-3893

243

Martial Arts America
1981 Hwy 54 West
Fayetteville, GA 30214
(770) 487-6464

ATA Karate Family Center
3940 Cherokee St., Suite #502
Kennesaw, GA 30144
(770) 427-8400

Droege's ATA Black Belt Academy
2800 Powder Springs Rd.
Marietta, GA 30064
(770) 222-1900

Fusion Martial Arts
1530 Old Alabama Rd., Suite 200
Roswell, GA 30076
(770) 992-7600

Statesboro Karate
199-A Northside Dr. East
Statesboro, GA 30458
(912) 764-5425

IDAHO
Idaho ATA Martial Arts
6025 W. Franklin Rd.
Boise, ID 83709
(208) 336-9750

Idaho ATA Martial Arts
1596 West Broadway
Idaho Falls, ID 83402
(208) 523-1161

ILLINOIS
Buffalo Grove Martial Arts
144 McHenry Rd.
Buffalo Grove IL 60089
(847) 215-8333

POW! Martial Arts Training School
950 West Washington St.
Chicago, IL 60607
(312) 829-7699

Ultimate Martial Arts Inc.
3922 W. Touhy Ave.
Lincolnwood, IL 60712
(847) 679-3330

INDIANA
Morris Dynamics
333 F Plaza East Blvd.
Evansville, IN 47715
(812) 471-8111

KANSAS
Krav Maga & Fitness Center
7844 Quivira Rd.
Lenexa, KS 66216
(913) 248-9696

KENTUCKY
Moberly's Black Belt Academies
501 Darby Creek Rd.
Lexington, KY 40507
(859) 264-1964

Core Modern Training Center
1920 Stanley Gault Parkway, Suite #200
Louisville, KY 40223
(502) 489-5444

LOUISIANA
Myers Family Karate Center
1010 C.M. Fagan Dr., #103
Hammond, LA 70403
(985) 542-7115

MARYLAND/ WASHINGTON, D.C.
Krav Maga Bowie
100 Whitemarsh Park Dr.
Bowie MD 20715
(571) 277-1927

Krav Maga Maryland-Columbia
8865 Stanford Blvd., Suite 141
Columbia, MD 21045
(410) 872-9194

Gordon's Self Defense Academy
13404 Kingsview Village Ave.
Germantown, MD 20874
(301) 972-5425

Krav Maga Maryland-Owings Mills
11299 Owings Mill Blvd., #113
Owings Mill, MD 21117
(410) 356-0707

Gordon's Self Defense Academy
1776 E. Jefferson St., #118
Rockville, MD 20850
(301) 972-5425

Krav Maga DC, Inc.
1716 Newton St. NW
Washington, DC 20010
(202) 332-0765

MASSACHUSETTS
America's Best Defense
171 Commonwealth Dr.
Attleboro Falls, MA 02763
(508) 699-0800

Krav Maga Boston
123 Terrace St.
Boston, MA 02120

Krav Maga Nantucket
150 Old South Rd.
Nantucket, MA 02554
(508) 325-5587

Fournier's Olympic Karate Center
1053 Forest Ave.
Portland, MA 04103
(207) 797-0900

245

MacDonald's Academy of Martial Arts
32 Arsenal St.
Watertown, MA 02472
(617) 923-4248

ATA Black Belt Academy
380 Middleset Ave.
Wilmington, MA 01887
(978) 658.6511

MICHIGAN
Ohana Family Karate and Fitness Center
7150 W. Grand River
Fowlerville, MI 48836
(517) 223-9131

West Side Self-Defense & Fitness
12330 James St., #110
Holland, MI 49424
(616) 394-5398

Krav Maga Detroit
4314 Rochester Rd.
Troy, MI 48084
(248) 643-4448

The Fighting Fit
4036 Biddle St.
Wyandotte, MI 48192
(734) 285-5875

MINNESOTA
Training for Life, Inc.
2748 Lyndale Ave.
South Minneapolis, MN 55408
(612) 871-0986

MISSOURI
Gateway Krav Maga, Inc.
12528 Olive Blvd., Suite D & E
Creve Coeur, MO 63141
(314) 205-1922

NEVADA
Brandon's Black Belt Academy & Karate for Kids
2549 Wigwam Pkwy
Henderson, NV 89014
(702) 897-7225

Contact Combat Systems, LLC
7925 W. Sahara Ave., Suite 103
Las Vegas, NV 89117
(702) 240-5166

NEBRASKA
Kassebaum's ATA Black Belt Academy
2111 Harvell Dr.
Bellevue, NE 68005
(402) 682-5425

Longoria's ATA Black Belt Academy
1432 N. Cottner Blvd.
Lincoln, NE 68505
(402) 466-2433

NEW HAMPSHIRE
Salem Self Defense Center
291 So. Broadway (Rt. 28)
Salem, NH 03079
(603) 890-3412

NEW JERSEY
Capobianco's Black Belt Academy
3 Lexington Ave.
East Brunswick, NJ 08816
(732) 257-5999

ATA Black Belt Academy
115 Stryker Lane, Suite 6 Bldg. 4
Hillsborough, NJ 08844
(908) 281-1800

NEW YORK
Top Gun Karate & Fitness
1170 Northern Blvd.
Manhasset, NY 11030
(516) 365-5382

KMLI – Self Defense & Fitness
21 West Nicholai Street
Hicksville, NY 11801
(516) 935-5728

Black Belt Academy
70 Union Avenue
Ronkonkoma, NY 11779
(631) 580-0686

Steve Sohn's Jujitsu Concepts
79 Montgomery Ave.
Scarsdale, NY 10583
(914) 723.7818

KM Northeast Regional Training Center
8200 Main St.
Williamsville, NY 14221
(716) 565-9568

Davide Yorktown Total Fitness
1761 Front St.
Yorktown Heights, NY 10598
(914) 302-7392

NORTH CAROLINA
ATA Black Belt Academy
3729 Sycamore Dairy Road, Suite 103
Fayetteville, NC 28303
(910) 860-5425

Ryan Hoover's Extreme Karate
1122 E. Hudson Blvd., Suite 1
Gastonia NC, 28054
(704) 867-4020

ATA Black Belt Academy
3515 Trent Rd.
New Bern, NC 28532
(910) 860-5425

OHIO

Core Tactix
6791 Dublin Center Dr.
Dublin, OH 43017
(614) 336-3780

Ohio Krav Maga Gahanna Tae Kwon Do Center
1000 Morrison Rd., Ste. #A
Gahana, OH 43085

Scott Gray Martial Art, Inc
10139 Royalton Rd., Suite C
N. Royalton, OH 44133
(440) 877-9108

The Black Belt Academy
148 E. South Boundary
Perrysburg, OH 43551
(419) 872-7599

OKLAHOMA

Krav Maga of Tulsa
3403 S. Peoria, #200
Tulsa, OK 74105
(918) 402-5800

OREGON

Turner's Tae Kwon Do, Inc.
1711 SE Hill St.
Albany, OR 97321
(541) 928-9636

Turner's Tae Kwon Do, Inc.
400 B South West 4th St.
Corvallis, OR 97330
(541) 752-3220

Krav Maga Oregon
121 West 6th Avenue
Junction City, OR 97448
(541) 998-6004

Krav Maga Self Defense & Fitness
4710 SW Scholls Ferry Rd.
Portland, OR 97225
(503) 297-7878

Koch Martial Arts
333 Main St.
Toledo, OR 97391
(541) 336-238

PENNSYLVANIA

Krav Maga Berwin
812 Lancaster
Berwin, PA 19382
(610) 647-6440

DeStolfo's Tae Kwon Do
1950 East Main Ave.
Conshohocken, PA 19428
(610) 834-8533

Kirk's Martial Arts Academy
1810 Wilmington Pike, Suite 12
Glenn Mills, PA 19342
(484) 880-2413

Kirk's Martial Arts Academy
826 E. Baltimore Pike Store #7
Kennette Square, PA 19348
(610) 444-8960

Lebanon Isshinryu Karate Inc.
970 Isabel Dr.
Lebanon, PA 17042
(717) 272-9890

SOUTH CAROLINA
Charleston Krav Maga
1017 Wappoo Rd.
Charleston, SC 29407

Charleston Krav Maga
4874 Marshwood
Hollywood, SC 29449
(843) 693-5425

TENNESSEE
Bullman's Boxing & Fitness
8079-0 Kingston Pike
Knoxville, TN 37919
(865) 470-8883

Mid-South Krav Maga
7193 Highway 64
Memphis, TN 38133
(901) 213-0933

Mid-South Krav Maga
2873 Poplar Ave.
Memphis, TN 38111
(901) 213-0933

TEXAS
Performance Fitness & Self Defense
1328 W. McDermott Dr., Suite 250
Allen, TX 75013
(469)939-1949

Black Belt Academy
4101 W. Green Oaks Blvd. #343
Arlington, TX 76016
(817) 478-5665

Fit and Fearless
118 E. Alpine Road
Austin, TX 78704
(512) 441-KRAV

Krav Maga Training Center
1901 W. William Cannon Dr #121
Austin, TX 78745
(512) 441-5728

Just Results, LLC
6829 Airport Blvd. #164
Austin, TX 78752
(512) 323-9070

Krav Maga Training Center
3601 South Congress Ave., Ste. G300
Austin, TX 78704
(512) 441-5728

Self Defense Texas LLC
12300 Riata Trace Parkway
Austin, TX 78727
(512) 310-0193

Tiger Clay's Mid-Cities Martial Arts
209 Bedford Rd., Suite 135
Bedford, TX 76022
(817) 282-3139

Sidekicks Martial Arts
2212 S. Market St. #122
Brenham, TX 77833
(979) 251-8824

Austing Self Defense, LLC
251 N. Bell, Ste. 108-A
Cedar Park, TX 78613
(512) 918-9999

Krav Maga Sidekicks
12845 Wellbourrn Rd., Ste. 120
College Station, TX 77845
(979) 694-1280

Personal Safety & Fitness Systems
4043 Trinity Mills, Suite 118
Dallas, TX 75287
(469) 667-3076

Krav Maga Houston
3930 Kirby Dr.
Houston, TX 77098
(832) 603-3473

Lakeway Elite Fitness
15006 Cavalier Canyon
Lakeway, TX 78734
(512) 968-8335

Al Garza's Martial Arts America
2047 West Main C-9
League City, TX 77573
(281) 332-5425

Self Defense Texas LLC
2401 Pecan Rm 1825
Pflugerville, TX
(512) 310-0193

Higher State Fitness
900 Round Rock Ave., Suite 212
Round Rock, TX 78681
(512) 310-2233

911 Self Defense, Inc
7460 Callaghan
San Antonio, TX 78229
(210) 348-6127

Just Results
1101 Thorpe Lane, Ste. C
San Marcos, TX 78666
(512) 392-5728

Krav Maga Victoria
5803 John Stockbauer Dr. Ste. C
Victoria, TX 77904
(361) 570-5728

UTAH
New Millennium Martial Arts
1450 South 400 West
Salt Lake City ,UT 84115-5109
(801) 563-3378

VIRGINIA
One Spirit Martial Arts, LLC
295 Sunset Park Dr
Herndon, VA 20170
(703)796-5508

Krav Maga Nova
8253 Backlick Rd #D
Lorton, VA 22079
(703) 339-0881

Wind & Sea Tae Kwon Do, Inc.
2253 W. Great Neck Rd.
Virginia Beach, VA 23451
(757) 496-3293

Thomas' Black Belt Academy III, Inc.
1169 Nimmo Prkwy, Unit 216
Virginia Beach, VA 23456
(757) 563-9022

Thomas' Black Belt Academy III, Inc.
3809 Princess Anne Rd., Suite #116
Virginia Beach, VA 23456
(757) 471-9002

JCC of South Hampton Road
3636 Virginia Beach Blvd
Virginia Beach, VA 23452
(757) 547-0508

WASHINGTON
Krav Maga East Side Training Center
13433 North East 20 St., Suite G
Bellevue, WA 98005
(425) 736-6019

Premier Martial Arts
12623 Meridian, Suite B
Puyallup, WA 98373
(253) 848-5425

East West Martial Arts
6204 NE Hwy 99
Vancouver, WA 98665
(360) 695-6845

WISCONSIN
Chay's Tae Kwon Do School
2720 Old Mill Dr
Racine, WI 53405
(262) 633-7090

Karate America
1700 East U.S. Hwy 14
Janesville, WI 53545
(608) 752-7283

Krav Maga-Milwaukee
17000 W. Capitol Dr
Brookfield, WI 53005
(262) 412-3757

251

APPENDIX B EXERCISES

INDEX

Abdominal muscles, 184, 187

Abraham, S. D., 4

Active-static stretching, 97, 99, 226–27

Activity, and caloric intake, 29–30

Activity, and flexibility, 47

Acute injuries, 124, 126

Adrenaline, 103

Advancing Left-Right Combo Drill, 213

Advancing Movements, 147–48

Advancing Straight Punch Drill, 212

Advancing Straight Punches, 152–53, 212

Aerobic exercise, 39–40, 61, 99, 118

Aerobic training, 39–40, 116–20

Age, and flexibility, 47

Agility, 174–76

Alternating Straight Punch Drill, 210–11

Anaerobic training, 116–20

Antioxidants, 30

Anxiety, 13, 14, 15

Associations, 237–49

Athletes, 29–30, 40, 62

Audible stimuli, 179, 216

Back muscles, 184–86

Back pain, 46, 183

Balance

and coordination, 75, 105–13

dynamic balance, 106–7, 110–11

improving, 105

and inner ear, 106

for kicking, 159–72

losing, 111

poses for, 108–9, 111

regaining, 112

static balance, 106–9

training for, 111–12

types of, 106–7

understanding, 106

and vision, 106

Bale, Christian, 10

Ball, medicine, 67, 76, 87–88, 134

Ball, weighted, 72, 87, 134, 222

Barak, Sheiki, xi

Base of support, 110

Basic fight combinations, 168–69, 227

Basic Squat, 66

Beginners

Fitness Format A, 199–203

Fitness Format B, 204–7

techniques for, 145–57, 199–207

tips for, 139–41, 172, 199

warm-ups for, 200–201

Ben-Asher, David, xi

261

263

Motor skills, 17, 43, 179, 213

Movement Stances, 147–48

Muay Thai kickboxing, 60

Multifidus muscle, 184

Muscle contraction rate, 93

Muscle cramps, 28, 30, 127

Muscle groups, 64

Muscle hypertrophy, 60

Muscle injury, 46–47, 60–61, 72, 126. *See also* Injuries

Muscle mass, 30, 61–62, 142

Muscle reactions, 60

Muscle soreness, 94, 102, 127, 200, 203

Muscle tissue, 126, 142

Muscle weight, 10

Muscular endurance, 63. *See also* Endurance

Muscular power, 73–85

Muscular strength, 59–72

Myocardial infarction, 98

Natural movements, 140

Nerve compression, 183

Nerve function, 93

Nervous system, 112, 140

Neutral Stance, 146

No-holds-barred (NHB), 7, 139

"No pain, no gain" myth, 94

Nutrients, 22, 27. *See also* Healthy eating

Nutrition, 12–13, 21–31, 34, 43

Obesity, 12

Obliques, 184

Olympic lifting, 88

One-repetition maximum (1-RM), 61

Organizations, 237–49

Osteoarthritis, 125

Overhead Rotations, 196

Overstretching, 46

Overtraining, 130

Oxygen consumption, 35–39, 93, 116

Pad holder, 151

Pain, 46, 94, 96, 124–29, 183

Partners, 233

Pelvic muscles, 184, 185

Perceived exertion, 42, 43

Perets, Amir, xi

Perseverance, 9

Phosphagen system, 117–18

Physical fitness, 34–35

Physiological warm-up, 92

Plank exercises, 188–89

Plateaus, 119

Platform Jump, 78

THE EVERYTHING SERIES!

BUSINESS & PERSONAL FINANCE

Everything® Accounting Book
Everything® Budgeting Book
Everything® Business Planning Book
Everything® Coaching and Mentoring Book
Everything® Fundraising Book
Everything® Get Out of Debt Book
Everything® Grant Writing Book
Everything® Guide to Personal Finance for Single Mothers
Everything® Home-Based Business Book, 2nd Ed.
Everything® Homebuying Book, 2nd Ed.
Everything® Homeselling Book, 2nd Ed.
Everything® Improve Your Credit Book
Everything® Investing Book, 2nd Ed.
Everything® Landlording Book
Everything® Leadership Book
Everything® Managing People Book, 2nd Ed.
Everything® Negotiating Book
Everything® Online Auctions Book
Everything® Online Business Book
Everything® Personal Finance Book
Everything® Personal Finance in Your 20s and 30s Book
Everything® Project Management Book
Everything® Real Estate Investing Book
Everything® Retirement Planning Book
Everything® Robert's Rules Book, $7.95
Everything® Selling Book
Everything® Start Your Own Business Book, 2nd Ed.
Everything® Wills & Estate Planning Book

COOKING

Everything® Barbecue Cookbook
Everything® Bartender's Book, $9.95
Everything® Cheese Book
Everything® Chinese Cookbook
Everything® Classic Recipes Book
Everything® Cocktail Parties and Drinks Book
Everything® College Cookbook
Everything® Cooking for Baby and Toddler Book
Everything® Cooking for Two Cookbook
Everything® Diabetes Cookbook
Everything® Easy Gourmet Cookbook
Everything® Fondue Cookbook
Everything® Fondue Party Book
Everything® Gluten-Free Cookbook
Everything® Glycemic Index Cookbook
Everything® Grilling Cookbook

Everything® Healthy Meals in Minutes Cookbook
Everything® Holiday Cookbook
Everything® Indian Cookbook
Everything® Italian Cookbook
Everything® Low-Carb Cookbook
Everything® Low-Fat High-Flavor Cookbook
Everything® Low-Salt Cookbook
Everything® Meals for a Month Cookbook
Everything® Mediterranean Cookbook
Everything® Mexican Cookbook
Everything® No Trans Fat Cookbook
Everything® One-Pot Cookbook
Everything® Pizza Cookbook
Everything® Quick and Easy 30-Minute, 5-Ingredient Cookbook
Everything® Quick Meals Cookbook
Everything® Slow Cooker Cookbook
Everything® Slow Cooking for a Crowd Cookbook
Everything® Soup Cookbook
Everything® Stir-Fry Cookbook
Everything® Tex-Mex Cookbook
Everything® Thai Cookbook
Everything® Vegetarian Cookbook
Everything® Wild Game Cookbook
Everything® Wine Book, 2nd Ed.

GAMES

Everything® 15-Minute Sudoku Book, $9.95
Everything® 30-Minute Sudoku Book, $9.95
Everything® Blackjack Strategy Book
Everything® Brain Strain Book, $9.95
Everything® Bridge Book
Everything® Card Games Book
Everything® Card Tricks Book, $9.95
Everything® Casino Gambling Book, 2nd Ed.
Everything® Chess Basics Book
Everything® Craps Strategy Book
Everything® Crossword and Puzzle Book
Everything® Crossword Challenge Book
Everything® Crosswords for the Beach Book, $9.95
Everything® Cryptograms Book, $9.95
Everything® Easy Crosswords Book
Everything® Easy Kakuro Book, $9.95
Everything® Easy Large Print Crosswords Book
Everything® Games Book, 2nd Ed.
Everything® Giant Sudoku Book, $9.95
Everything® Kakuro Challenge Book, $9.95
Everything® Large-Print Crossword Challenge Book
Everything® Large-Print Crosswords Book

Everything® Lateral Thinking Puzzles Book, $9.95
Everything® Mazes Book
Everything® Movie Crosswords Book, $9.95
Everything® Online Poker Book, $12.95
Everything® Pencil Puzzles Book, $9.95
Everything® Poker Strategy Book
Everything® Pool & Billiards Book
Everything® Sports Crosswords Book, $9.95
Everything® Test Your IQ Book, $9.95
Everything® Texas Hold 'Em Book, $9.95
Everything® Travel Crosswords Book, $9.95
Everything® Word Games Challenge Book
Everything® Word Scramble Book
Everything® Word Search Book

HEALTH

Everything® Alzheimer's Book
Everything® Diabetes Book
Everything® Health Guide to Adult Bipolar Disorder
Everything® Health Guide to Controlling Anxiety
Everything® Health Guide to Fibromyalgia
Everything® Health Guide to Postpartum Care
Everything® Health Guide to Thyroid Disease
Everything® Hypnosis Book
Everything® Low Cholesterol Book
Everything® Massage Book
Everything® Menopause Book
Everything® Nutrition Book
Everything® Reflexology Book
Everything® Stress Management Book

HISTORY

Everything® American Government Book
Everything® American History Book, 2nd Ed.
Everything® Civil War Book
Everything® Freemasons Book
Everything® Irish History & Heritage Book
Everything® Middle East Book

HOBBIES

Everything® Candlemaking Book
Everything® Cartooning Book
Everything® Coin Collecting Book
Everything® Drawing Book
Everything® Family Tree Book, 2nd Ed.
Everything® Knitting Book
Everything® Knots Book
Everything® Photography Book
Everything® Quilting Book
Everything® Scrapbooking Book

Everything® Sewing Book
Everything® Soapmaking Book, 2nd Ed.
Everything® Woodworking Book

HOME IMPROVEMENT

Everything® Feng Shui Book
Everything® Feng Shui Decluttering Book, $9.95
Everything® Fix-It Book
Everything® Home Decorating Book
Everything® Home Storage Solutions Book
Everything® Homebuilding Book
Everything® Organize Your Home Book

KIDS' BOOKS

All titles are $7.95

Everything® Kids' Animal Puzzle & Activity Book
Everything® Kids' Baseball Book, 4th Ed.
Everything® Kids' Bible Trivia Book
Everything® Kids' Bugs Book
Everything® Kids' Cars and Trucks Puzzle
   & Activity Book
Everything® Kids' Christmas Puzzle
   & Activity Book
Everything® Kids' Cookbook
Everything® Kids' Crazy Puzzles Book
Everything® Kids' Dinosaurs Book
Everything® Kids' First Spanish Puzzle and
   Activity Book
Everything® Kids' Gross Cookbook
Everything® Kids' Gross Hidden Pictures Book
Everything® Kids' Gross Jokes Book
Everything® Kids' Gross Mazes Book
Everything® Kids' Gross Puzzle and
   Activity Book
Everything® Kids' Halloween Puzzle
   & Activity Book
Everything® Kids' Hidden Pictures Book
Everything® Kids' Horses Book
Everything® Kids' Joke Book
Everything® Kids' Knock Knock Book
Everything® Kids' Learning Spanish Book
Everything® Kids' Math Puzzles Book
Everything® Kids' Mazes Book
Everything® Kids' Money Book
Everything® Kids' Nature Book
Everything® Kids' Pirates Puzzle and Activity Book
Everything® Kids' Presidents Book
Everything® Kids' Princess Puzzle and Activity Book
Everything® Kids' Puzzle Book
Everything® Kids' Riddles & Brain Teasers Book
Everything® Kids' Science Experiments Book
Everything® Kids' Sharks Book
Everything® Kids' Soccer Book
Everything® Kids' States Book
Everything® Kids' Travel Activity Book

KIDS' STORY BOOKS

Everything® Fairy Tales Book

LANGUAGE

Everything® Conversational Japanese Book with
   CD, $19.95
Everything® French Grammar Book
Everything® French Phrase Book, $9.95
Everything® French Verb Book, $9.95
Everything® German Practice Book with CD,
   $19.95
Everything® Inglés Book
Everything® Intermediate Spanish Book with
   CD, $19.95
Everything® Learning Brazilian Portuguese
   Book with CD, $19.95
Everything® Learning French Book
Everything® Learning German Book
Everything® Learning Italian Book
Everything® Learning Latin Book
Everything® Learning Spanish Book with CD,
   2nd Edition, $19.95
Everything® Russian Practice Book with CD,
   $19.95
Everything® Sign Language Book
Everything® Spanish Grammar Book
Everything® Spanish Phrase Book, $9.95
Everything® Spanish Practice Book
   with CD, $19.95
Everything® Spanish Verb Book, $9.95
Everything® Speaking Mandarin Chinese Book
   with CD, $19.95

MUSIC

Everything® Drums Book with CD, $19.95
Everything® Guitar Book with CD, 2nd Edition,
   $19.95
Everything® Guitar Chords Book with CD, $19.95
Everything® Home Recording Book
Everything® Music Theory Book with CD, $19.95
Everything® Reading Music Book with CD, $19.95
Everything® Rock & Blues Guitar Book
   with CD, $19.95
Everything® Rock and Blues Piano Book with
   CD, $19.95
Everything® Songwriting Book

NEW AGE

Everything® Astrology Book, 2nd Ed.
Everything® Birthday Personology Book
Everything® Dreams Book, 2nd Ed.
Everything® Love Signs Book, $9.95
Everything® Numerology Book
Everything® Paganism Book
Everything® Palmistry Book
Everything® Psychic Book
Everything® Reiki Book
Everything® Sex Signs Book, $9.95

Everything® Tarot Book, 2nd Ed.
Everything® Toltec Wisdom Book
Everything® Wicca and Witchcraft Book

PARENTING

Everything® Baby Names Book, 2nd Ed.
Everything® Baby Shower Book
Everything® Baby's First Year Book
Everything® Birthing Book
Everything® Breastfeeding Book
Everything® Father-to-Be Book
Everything® Father's First Year Book
Everything® Get Ready for Baby Book
Everything® Get Your Baby to Sleep Book, $9.95
Everything® Getting Pregnant Book
Everything® Guide to Raising a One-Year-Old
Everything® Guide to Raising a Two-Year-Old
Everything® Homeschooling Book
Everything® Mother's First Year Book
Everything® Parent's Guide to Childhood
   Illnesses
Everything® Parent's Guide to Children
   and Divorce
Everything® Parent's Guide to Children
   with ADD/ADHD
Everything® Parent's Guide to Children
   with Asperger's Syndrome
Everything® Parent's Guide to Children
   with Autism
Everything® Parent's Guide to Children with
   Bipolar Disorder
Everything® Parent's Guide to Children with
   Depression
Everything® Parent's Guide to Children
   with Dyslexia
Everything® Parent's Guide to Children with
   Juvenile Diabetes
Everything® Parent's Guide to Positive Discipline
Everything® Parent's Guide to Raising a
   Successful Child
Everything® Parent's Guide to Raising Boys
Everything® Parent's Guide to Raising Girls
Everything® Parent's Guide to Raising Siblings
Everything® Parent's Guide to Sensory
   Integration Disorder
Everything® Parent's Guide to Tantrums
Everything® Parent's Guide to the Strong-Willed
   Child
Everything® Parenting a Teenager Book
Everything® Potty Training Book, $9.95
Everything® Pregnancy Book, 3rd Ed.
Everything® Pregnancy Fitness Book
Everything® Pregnancy Nutrition Book
Everything® Pregnancy Organizer, 2nd Ed.,
   $16.95
Everything® Toddler Activities Book
Everything® Toddler Book

Everything® Tween Book
Everything® Twins, Triplets, and More Book

PETS

Everything® Aquarium Book
Everything® Boxer Book
Everything® Cat Book, 2nd Ed.
Everything® Chihuahua Book
Everything® Dachshund Book
Everything® Dog Book
Everything® Dog Health Book
Everything® Dog Obedience Book
Everything® Dog Owner's Organizer, $16.95
Everything® Dog Training and Tricks Book
Everything® German Shepherd Book
Everything® Golden Retriever Book
Everything® Horse Book
Everything® Horse Care Book
Everything® Horseback Riding Book
Everything® Labrador Retriever Book
Everything® Poodle Book
Everything® Pug Book
Everything® Puppy Book
Everything® Rottweiler Book
Everything® Small Dogs Book
Everything® Tropical Fish Book
Everything® Yorkshire Terrier Book

REFERENCE

Everything® American Presidents Book
Everything® Blogging Book
Everything® Build Your Vocabulary Book
Everything® Car Care Book
Everything® Classical Mythology Book
Everything® Da Vinci Book
Everything® Divorce Book
Everything® Einstein Book
Everything® Enneagram Book
Everything® Etiquette Book, 2nd Ed.
Everything® Inventions and Patents Book
Everything® Mafia Book
Everything® Philosophy Book
Everything® Pirates Book
Everything® Psychology Book

RELIGION

Everything® Angels Book
Everything® Bible Book
Everything® Buddhism Book
Everything® Catholicism Book
Everything® Christianity Book
Everything® Gnostic Gospels Book
Everything® History of the Bible Book
Everything® Jesus Book

Everything® Jewish History & Heritage Book
Everything® Judaism Book
Everything® Kabbalah Book
Everything® Koran Book
Everything® Mary Book
Everything® Mary Magdalene Book
Everything® Prayer Book
Everything® Saints Book, 2nd Ed.
Everything® Torah Book
Everything® Understanding Islam Book
Everything® World's Religions Book
Everything® Zen Book

SCHOOL & CAREERS

Everything® Alternative Careers Book
Everything® Career Tests Book
Everything® College Major Test Book
Everything® College Survival Book, 2nd Ed.
Everything® Cover Letter Book, 2nd Ed.
Everything® Filmmaking Book
Everything® Get-a-Job Book, 2nd Ed.
Everything® Guide to Being a Paralegal
Everything® Guide to Being a Personal Trainer
Everything® Guide to Being a Real Estate Agent
Everything® Guide to Being a Sales Rep
Everything® Guide to Careers in Health Care
Everything® Guide to Careers in Law Enforcement
Everything® Guide to Government Jobs
Everything® Guide to Starting and Running a Restaurant
Everything® Job Interview Book
Everything® New Nurse Book
Everything® New Teacher Book
Everything® Paying for College Book
Everything® Practice Interview Book
Everything® Resume Book, 2nd Ed.
Everything® Study Book

SELF-HELP

Everything® Dating Book, 2nd Ed.
Everything® Great Sex Book
Everything® Self-Esteem Book
Everything® Tantric Sex Book

SPORTS & FITNESS

Everything® Easy Fitness Book
Everything® Running Book
Everything® Weight Training Book

TRAVEL

Everything® Family Guide to Cruise Vacations
Everything® Family Guide to Hawaii
Everything® Family Guide to Las Vegas, 2nd Ed.
Everything® Family Guide to Mexico
Everything® Family Guide to New York City, 2nd Ed.
Everything® Family Guide to RV Travel & Campgrounds
Everything® Family Guide to the Caribbean
Everything® Family Guide to the Walt Disney World Resort®, Universal Studios®, and Greater Orlando, 4th Ed.
Everything® Family Guide to Timeshares
Everything® Family Guide to Washington D.C., 2nd Ed.

WEDDINGS

Everything® Bachelorette Party Book, $9.95
Everything® Bridesmaid Book, $9.95
Everything® Destination Wedding Book
Everything® Elopement Book, $9.95
Everything® Father of the Bride Book, $9.95
Everything® Groom Book, $9.95
Everything® Mother of the Bride Book, $9.95
Everything® Outdoor Wedding Book
Everything® Wedding Book, 3rd Ed.
Everything® Wedding Checklist, $9.95
Everything® Wedding Etiquette Book, $9.95
Everything® Wedding Organizer, 2nd Ed., $16.95
Everything® Wedding Shower Book, $9.95
Everything® Wedding Vows Book, $9.95
Everything® Wedding Workout Book
Everything® Weddings on a Budget Book, $9.95

WRITING

Everything® Creative Writing Book
Everything® Get Published Book, 2nd Ed.
Everything® Grammar and Style Book
Everything® Guide to Magazine Writing
Everything® Guide to Writing a Book Proposal
Everything® Guide to Writing a Novel
Everything® Guide to Writing Children's Books
Everything® Guide to Writing Copy
Everything® Guide to Writing Research Papers
Everything® Screenwriting Book
Everything® Writing Poetry Book
Everything® Writing Well Book